CW01509935

In a culture saturated with sexualized content but lacking real conversations about intimacy and sexual health, Drs. Stephanie Covington and Vanessa Carlisle offer a powerful, insightful master class on embracing our sexuality and reconnecting with our authentic selves in recovery.

Candice Norcott, PhD, licensed clinical psychologist, associate professor, and clinical director of the Obstetrics & Gynecology Mental Health Program at the University of Chicago

◦ ◉ ◦

As a woman in long-term recovery, I know how often our bodies, sexuality, and pleasure are left out of the healing conversation. *Awaken Your Sexuality* is a brave and necessary invitation to reclaim what addiction, trauma, or shame may have silenced. It speaks directly to our lived experience and centers intimacy—not just sex—as essential to recovery. The authors remind us that recovery can hold all of who we are—and that pleasure, connection, and belonging are ours to claim.

Dawn Nickel, PhD, founder of SHE RECOVERS Foundation

◦ ◉ ◦

Awaken Your Sexuality puts women and nonbinary people at the center of a topic that too often leaves us out: how to thrive as a sexually authentic and vibrant human being, no matter the specifics. Through thought-provoking questions, personal stories, cultural analysis, and practical exercises, Covington and Carlisle guide readers through a gentle, powerful, and healing path of sexual self-discovery.

August McLaughlin, author, journalist, and host/producer of *Girl Boner Radio*

◦ ◉ ◦

Stephanie Covington and Vanessa Carlisle's book *Awaken Your Sexuality: A Guide to Connection and Intimacy After Addiction and Trauma* gives the reader tips and stories that explore the sexual and sensual self—especially for those who experienced childhood sexual abuse or adult sexual assault—and that reclaim the inner self and integrate with the outer world. This book nurtures the reader to empower a sense of sexual self-awareness and authenticity. Becoming self-compassionate in one's own recovery is essential. For this survivor of childhood sexual abuse who has moved to being a sexual thriver, this book is a positive guide that promotes a lifelong journey to enjoy!

Cynthia Moreno Tuohy, BSW, NCAC II, CDC III, SAP,
immediate past executive director and past president
of NAADAC, author of *Rein In Your Brain: From
Impulsivity to Thoughtful Living in Recovery*

○ ● ○

Awaken Your Sexuality is the book I needed when I was newly sober, and it still helps me after ten years of recovery. Covington and Carlisle have an inclusive insight that brings nuance to the intersection of trauma and intimacy.

Tawny Lara, author of *Dry Humping: A Guide to Dating,
Relating, and Hooking Up Without the Booze*

○ ● ○

Awaken Your Sexuality is a wise, gentle guide for women on the path of sexual recovery. Bolstered by decades of research and grounded in lived experience, Covington and Carlisle welcome readers into a transformational process of self-reflection. Everyone will recognize parts of themself in the collected stories of women and nonbinary people who have developed self-compassion and learned to embrace their own pleasure. With helpful exercises and plenty of encouragement along the way, this book is a must-read for all of us who want deeper connection and intimacy in our sexual lives.

Lisa Cypers Kamen, MA, Adv. CASAC, CADC II,
Harvesting Happiness Lifestyle Management Consulting

○ ◎ ○

Drs. Covington and Carlisle guide their reader through reconnection to self while deconstructing systemic myths and increasing survivors' hope and pleasure. This book is a needed tool for anyone exploring connections between sexuality, healing, and recovery.

Theodore Burnes, PhD, professor of Clinical
Education and licensed clinical psychologist
at the University of Southern California

○ ◎ ○

Covington and Carlisle balance honest explorations of harmful sexual history and seeking sexual safety with an invitation to explore sexual pleasures. *Awaken Your Sexuality* is essential reading given the slumbering state of American substance use programs yet to wake up and become curious about the rich and essential sexual lives of the people they treat.

Douglas Braun-Harvey, MFT, CST-S,
co-founder of The Harvey Institute

Awaken
YOUR SEXUALITY

A Guide to Connection and Intimacy
after Addiction and Trauma

STEPHANIE S. COVINGTON, PhD, LCSW
VANESSA CARLISLE, PhD

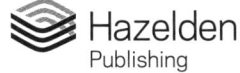

Hazelden
Publishing

Hazelden Publishing
Center City, Minnesota 55012
hazelden.org/bookstore

ISBN: 978-1-63634-092-0
Ebook ISBN: 978-1-63634-094-4

Library of Congress Cataloging-in-Publication Data is on file with the Library
of Congress.

Editor's notes
Hazelden Publishing offers a variety of information on addiction and related
areas. Our publications do not necessarily represent Hazelden Betty Ford Foundation's programs, nor do they officially speak for any Twelve Step organization.

The stories shared in this book were used with the consent of the individuals involved.

Readers should be aware that websites listed in this work may have changed
or disappeared between when this work was written and when it is read.

29 28 27 26 25   1 2 3 4 5 6

Art Director: Terri Kinne
Cover and interior design: Sara Streifel, Think Creative Design
Developmental editor: Andy Lien
Production editor: Betty Christiansen

Dedicated to the clients, colleagues,
friends, and loved ones who have
courageously shared their stories
and experiences with us.

CONTENTS

CHAPTER 12

The Continuing Journey of
Sexual Recovery

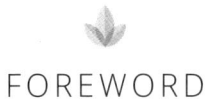

FOREWORD

A few years ago, I was invited to give a speech at a conference in Chicago called She Recovers—a wonderful gathering of women and nonbinary people from all corners of the addiction and recovery worlds.

I was fortunate enough to be seated at dinner next to a woman named Dr. Stephanie Covington, who was being honored that evening for her years of tireless work on behalf of female, transgender, and nonbinary addicts—particularly within the prison system. In the recovery circles in which I travel, Stephanie is something of a revered hero (most well known for her brilliant book *A Woman's Way Through the Twelve Steps*, which has helped many a friend of mine get sober). It was incredibly moving for me to get to meet someone whose work has been so important over the years to countless thousands of recovering addicts, and it was gratifying to see her receive not only a well-deserved award of honor, but also the love and gratitude of every single person in that room.

Stephanie and I immediately hit it off, and we spent the evening talking about our shared passion for addiction recovery and advocacy, and sharing bits of our own personal struggles and victories. After she heard my speech (in which I spoke openly about my history of sex and love addiction and the serenity I have found through the Twelve Steps), she mentioned that she and her co-writer, Vanessa Carlisle, were working on a book together about healthy sexuality within the context of recovery from addiction and trauma.

As Stephanie told me more about the project, I became increasingly intrigued. I knew immediately that this book was bound to become a treasured resource—especially for women, queer folk, and trans people (so many of whom have suffered and struggled to find safe, honest, and pleasurable pathways for their own sexual expression despite abuse, neglect, exploitation, oppression, lack of information, and the cruel and distorted messaging of their parents, their churches, the mass media, and, of course, the patriarchy). So many of us have been harmed and misled by our families and our culture that it reminds me of a line from a Simon & Garfunkel song: "I don't know a soul who's not been battered / I don't have a friend who feels at ease."

Who among us indeed feels at ease—and how do we find our way to satisfaction and peace?

"We need this book *yesterday*!" I told Stephanie, immediately thinking of all my recovery sisters, fellows, and sponsees who could benefit from just such a text. She just laughed and said that I might have to wait a while for it, but that the book was definitely coming.

Well, now the book is here—and it is even richer and more comprehensive than I could have dreamed.

The book you hold in your hands is not only about addiction and sexual trauma (although those two subjects are covered in thorough, thoughtful, and deeply intelligent detail); it's also about pleasure. It's about our *right* to pleasure—no matter what we have done in the past or what has been done to us. It's about the honesty, safety, experimentation, and transparency that we deserve to experience, both within our relationships and within our own private psyches. It's about how to set boundaries, how to understand what assault and abuse do to us on a physical and psychological level, how to *feel*, and how to be sexual while sober—perhaps for the first time in our lives, or at least in recent memory. It's about getting to define (and redefine) sensuality, intimacy, and commitment in any way that feels accurate to your own mind, body, and spirit.

I also love that this book pays homage to so many different ways of being, living, and feeling. The authors respectfully discuss monogamy, polyamory, divorce, sexual anorexia, sex work, hetero and queer sex, bisexuality, the sensual experiences of people with disabilities, bigger bodies, and aging bodies. They even discuss my current favorite sexual topic: how to find erotic fulfillment without a partner.

Nobody is judged in these pages; everyone is welcomed, and everyone is understood.

And oh, how deeply that understanding is needed—for all of us!

The authors present a beautiful definition of *addiction* in these pages, and one that I had never heard before. They call addiction "the chronic neglect of self in favor of something or someone else." They go on to explain that—long before we learned how to neglect ourselves—we were all too often neglected and abused by others. Where else would we have learned to treat ourselves so poorly? And why wouldn't that lack of self-respect translate into sexual suffering, confusion, and acting out? They write, "Sometimes we get so lost in being sexual the way our partner wants us to, or the way we were taught we should, or the way we've seen in movies or shows, or the only way we know how, that we aren't able to sense what brings us our own true pleasure. When we perform sexually for others more than we authentically engage with our body's likes and dislikes, we can get lost and out of balance."

And once you add mind-altering substances to the mix, or harmful compulsive behaviors, a person can become even *more* lost, and even *more* out of balance.

Yet hope is to be found, both within these pages and in our own recovery journeys.

What I appreciate most about this book is how careful the authors are to constantly bring the discussion back to *your* body, to *your* preferences, to *your* desires and needs and curiosities and hopes. When I work with newcomers in Twelve Step recovery, I often tell them that there are as many ways to get sober as there were to get high, and as many styles of recovery as there are people getting well. No one person has all the answers for another—and this book honors that truth with rare delicacy. We are reminded in these pages that there is no such thing as sexual "normalcy" and that we can change our minds and our behaviors as many times as we need to change in order to find our true selves. Furthermore, there is no gold standard that we must reach in order to become "good at sex," nor is there any bodily goal that we must achieve before we are allowed access to pleasure. No—we can awaken to the miracle of ourselves right here, right now, in this current form, in this current moment.

What a balm to see this message of self-acceptance and sacred inclusion—especially within the context of recovery. I am a member of *all* the Twelve Step programs that deal with relationship issues, and after years of sitting in rooms filled with my fellow codependents, chronic enablers, toxic self-abandoners, desperate people-pleasers, emotional anorexics, and those who have given themselves away more times than they can count, I have come to one conclusion.

The solution always seems to be: *Put the focus on yourself.*

This is how we get well.

Put the focus on yourself.

To learn how to feel our own feelings, to find our own opinions, to express our own desires, and to speak with our own voice—this is what recovery looks like. And this book shows you how to find that agency, that dignity, that literal ownership of yourself—within your ongoing recovery, and within the specific details of your own holy life.

I want to say one more thing, before you turn the page and embark upon this sacred journey at your own pace. (And please—with reading as with sex, always do move at your own pace!) I admire the fact that both Stephanie and Vanessa decided to include details from their own addiction histories and sexual experiences in these pages. They didn't need to do that, but they decided to do it. This choice seems both rare and fair to me—that the authors of a book about intimacy and addiction would be so revealing of themselves, rather than looking at the subject analytically, from the safe, cold, and outside position of "experts." That level of candid disclosure and sisterhood is exactly what I love most about the recovery process. None of us can get well in isolation, and nobody in this field should ever present themselves as an expert. You are the only expert on your own body, after all. How much more healing it is when everyone shares equally of their own experience, strength, and hope—without anyone telling anybody else what is right or wrong. We are all here to hold up lanterns for each other, as we each find our way.

Moved by the openness of the authors, I volunteered to be interviewed for this project, as well. It's an honor to have part of my story told here, interwoven with the experiences of so many others.

In other words, I'm happy not only to endorse this book, but to be part of it.

May you be safe, friends.

May you be well, may you be happy, and may you know peace and pleasure.

Most of all, may you know yourself.

—*Elizabeth Gilbert*

Now Is the Time

This book is for you if any of the following are true:

- You are doing some form of recovery: You may have experienced a substance use disorder, an eating disorder, or compulsive or addictive behaviors with spending, gambling, screen time, self-harm, work, relationships, sex, or anything else that caused harm to yourself or your loved ones. You have reached a point where you know that recovering sexually is also important for your well-being.

- It seems like it has been a long time since you felt genuine sexual pleasure, or maybe you never have.

- As a child, you felt afraid to ask questions about sex or gender because it seemed like there could be negative consequences. As an adult, you feel avoidant or nervous talking about sexuality.

- You have survived sexual trauma: sexual abuse, sexual assault, rape, or any other form of sexual violence, including workplace sexual harassment.

- You aren't comfortable having sexual contact without alcohol or another substance.

- Sex with your partner(s) often doesn't feel good or gives you intrusive thoughts and/or memories.

- You haven't had a sexual partner since you started recovering, and you are nervous to try again.

- You have been in a relationship that diminished your self-worth and made you feel undesirable.
- Your solo sex, or masturbation, is unsatisfying. You may avoid touching and exploring your own body.

This book is for all kinds of women who have survived something difficult and want to feel better. We will center on the experiences of women and nonbinary people who have lived through trauma, are recovering from harmful forms of substance use or compulsive behaviors, and are seeking a new, authentic connection to their sexuality.

Many of us have used substances to numb emotional pain from traumatic experiences. Many of us have stayed distracted from our pain by engaging in behaviors that get out of control and end up causing us more harm.

A trauma may be a singular event, such as a sexual assault, or it may be a series of pressures over time, such as the toxic stress associated with experiencing racism, not having enough money to meet basic needs, living in a body that doesn't conform to what's considered "normal," or growing up in an environment where girls, women, and nonbinary, transgender, and gender-expansive people are treated as less important than the cisgender boys and men around them.

We all need coping mechanisms to stay alive when the world around us discourages our essential human existence. Some of our coping mechanisms are nourishing and supportive to us, while others may give us temporary relief but contribute to our suffering in the long term. Recovery involves a transition from destructive coping habits to more positive ones. This is rarely something we do totally alone. We all need connection and belonging to make these changes.

You choose to awaken your sexuality because you are ready to experience the fullness of life. It happens to you when you decide you are ready to enjoy the creativity and pleasure of your unique body. That time can be now.

While we will feature the stories of women and nonbinary people who are recovering from addiction and trauma in this book, you do not have to be struggling with substance use to recognize the issues we discuss. Every woman and gender-expansive person living under patriarchy is recovering from something.

Part of connecting to your sexuality is encountering the way you think and feel about your gender and your body. Another part is how you want to be seen, felt, and known.

Our intended audience is anyone who identifies with the word *woman*. We welcome cisgender women, transgender women, nonbinary individuals who resonate with the experiences and challenges of women, and those who may not yet have labels or prefer no labels.

Gender and sexuality exist on their own spectrums, and variety is the most normal thing in the world. Heterosexual women, bisexual women, lesbian women, pansexual women, and queer, questioning, and asexual women will all find themselves represented in this book.

What we all have in common is the way our society was not designed to encourage our full, safe, creative, and enthusiastic participation. This reality persists despite the many gains women's and queer movements for rights and liberation have made over the decades.

Another word to notice is *addiction*. Both co-authors and many of our clients and friends use this word easily from their own experience, and it is still often used in institutional settings.

"Addiction medicine" is a growing field, and most treatment centers, rehabilitation facilities, and recovery groups use the term, even if they also use *substance use disorder* (SUD) and *alcohol use disorder* (AUD).

Many people also use the word *addiction* or *process addiction* to refer to out-of-control behaviors. These are behaviors that are not substance related, such as disordered eating, out-of-control gambling, compulsive spending, and so on. Current research is teasing out the complexity among these experiences. Our stories are getting told more and more. Still, the treatment options all look essentially the same.

Another distinction is usually drawn between addiction and compulsion. For example, compulsive handwashing associated with obsessive-compulsive disorder (OCD) is seen as quite different from the sense of overwhelming need one might feel to drink alcohol after becoming alcohol-dependent.

Some prefer to avoid the words *addiction* and also *sobriety* entirely. In harm reduction circles, abstinence from substances is not required for clients to receive treatment and care. Harm reduction philosophy offers strategies to reduce the negative consequences associated with substance use without mandating total sobriety or identification with the term *addiction*.

These conversations and distinctions are important. At the same time, they often lack a key piece of information: A large percentage of women who develop addictions and compulsive behaviors, including those associated with OCD and other mental health conditions such as anxiety and depression, are survivors of trauma. Trauma is often at the root of it all.

Throughout this book, we will use a variety of terms to refer to substance use disorders and compulsive or addictive behaviors. We intend to convey both the complexity of these experiences and the important features they share. We aim to use the language that is clearest, most descriptive, most true to the people represented, and least stigmatizing.

Overall, the definition of *addiction* we use is "chronic neglect of self in favor of something or someone else."

Context is critical: Some terms are more appropriate for speaking of significant trends among many people, and other terms reflect the individual experience of the person speaking. As terminology changes, we need to update our conversations to reflect it. We hope our language helps you feel seen and included, even when we discuss an experience you may not have had personally.

Why awaken your sexuality in the first place? If you have been frightened, confused, ashamed, or disconnected from your sexual self for a long time, feeling your own pleasure in a safe way may seem impossible. We assure you it is not. Our goal is to help you feel more pleasure and connection more often, in a way that supports and sustains you, with or without a partner.

Your relationship to your own body, pleasure, and sexuality has everything to do with your recovery, your relationships with the people in your life, and your ability to continue building the life you want. An intimate relationship with yourself creates the foundation for intimacy with others. Taking the time and doing this work allows you to heal pain from the past and feel more whole in the present.

Remember: The first step toward change is awareness. We can change only those things in our lives that we are aware of.

This book may serve as validation for what you have already come to know and feel, and as you read you may feel affirmed and more empowered. Or you may find that you need to read slowly and digest the material piece by piece because it stirs up painful memories and challenges your beliefs. We hope this book will suggest new ideas, highlight aspects of your own life that need attention, and open up entirely new understandings of your body, your pleasure, and your connections with others.

By reading *Awaken Your Sexuality*, you are choosing to become conscious about and connected to your authentic, unique sexuality as it exists in the present. As you become more connected to your sexuality, which includes your body's feelings and your emotional needs, you are also renewing the personal power of conscious choice. This will transform all your relationships, whether they are sexual partnerships or not.

Throughout the following pages, we will discuss the value of being in a therapeutic group that reflects your experience, such as a group for sexual assault survivors, a group for people recovering from eating disorders, a grief support group, or a recovery group for people who struggle with alcohol and other substance use. We encourage you to also seek a community as you do the private exploration of your sexuality addressed here. While Alcoholics Anonymous and associated Twelve Step groups are the most widely known, we recognize that there are as many paths to health as there are people, and we do not promote any particular program.

You will decide on your version of health and wholeness. Only you will know if you need to pursue therapy, medication, a dance class, a diploma, inpatient care, acupuncture, cultural ceremony, or any other modality. Most of us find we need a combination of resources, and some of them must be ongoing practices. Recovery does require time and effort. Sexual recovery may bring you new and different challenges, and setting aside time each day or week to engage with this material will serve you well.

Women and gender-expansive people experience harm due to sexism, misogyny, gender violence, homophobia, and transphobia. We believe that the reclamation of our diverse bodies, genders, and sexualities is a key component of our well-being and a step toward greater safety for all.

This book intends to help you connect with your unique sexuality through the stories of others. A content note: We will discuss vulvas and other female anatomy, the socialization of people assigned female at birth, and the experiences of girls and women, including nonbinary people and transgender women, both social and sexual. Some of these experiences are very painful, and others are hopeful and pleasurable, offering openings for your own growth.

The stories included here come from women and nonbinary people we have known personally, worked with in therapy and coaching, and encountered over our combined years. We have changed details, timelines, and names to protect individual identities, and we have created composites from real women's experiences to help illuminate common concerns and pathways forward.

What we offer here is a gentle exploration of the ways sexuality can be a positive force in your life. In part 1, you will get reacquainted with your body, your feelings, and your memories, and you will consciously engage with your experience of desire and pleasure. In part 2, you will revisit your history and gain deeper understanding of how your sexual self has come to be and what changes you are making now. In part 3, you will practice articulating what you want, like, and dislike and explore your current beliefs and values about sex, all with an eye toward your own pleasure. In part 4, you will develop the skills of connection and intimacy, with yourself and others. If you would like to take your exploration further, you can choose to complete the *Awaken Your Sexuality Workbook* in tandem with or after reading this book, whether in a group or on your own. We will suggest many other resources along the way.

Recovery is about living life fully and completely, and your sexual recovery is integral to the fullness of your life. While struggling with compulsive behaviors, problem use of a substance, or the symptoms of trauma (such as depression, anxiety, dissociation, and others), you likely have felt isolated and abandoned at times. In choosing to acknowledge and awaken your sexuality, you are embarking on an inner journey to reconnect with your best friend: your embodied self.

The same world that causes us harm is also filled with wonder and mystery. Your unique sexuality is powerful and can bring you joy, pleasure, and deeper trust in yourself. It doesn't happen overnight, but it is absolutely worth the effort.

○ ◉ ○

PART

1

Feelings: The Inner Journey

Being together sexually is a way for people to do any number of things: get close, bond, connect, avoid loneliness, have fun, play, interrupt boredom, fulfill a duty . . . the list goes on. But when our sexuality is defined or influenced by guilt, shame, trauma, or addiction, expressions of sexuality can feel disconnected from our desires and feelings.

Each of us has an inner life and an outer life. Our inner life is who we are and how we feel inside; our outer life is how we interact with others. When we live in active addiction or are consumed by the pain of trauma, our inner and outer lives are out of balance. We don't always act on our feelings, and often we don't even know what our feelings are. We may be suffering so profoundly we cannot experience our full range of feeling. Part of recovery is getting our inner lives and our outer lives to reflect more of each other, and to experience a wider range of feelings.

How well do you know your sexual self today? When was the last time you honestly examined your beliefs or assumptions about what you need and what you want? What are you thinking about when you look at your body in the mirror? What do you know about how your genitals look and feel? What is your range of sexual response? Many people have not deeply explored their beliefs and assumptions about their bodies, their sexual activities, their erotic selves, and their capacity for pleasure.

There are many reasons why we may choose not to focus on these questions, but there are two reasons that arise most often. The first is that it doesn't feel *safe* to awaken our sexuality. Second is that the reward for paying attention to our sexuality is not obvious or guaranteed. In other words, it's too scary or it isn't worth the trouble.

As a child, do you remember playing on the monkey bars? In order to swing and move ahead, you had to let go of the bar behind so that you could reach out to the next. There was a moment when you were holding on to nothing. The momentum of moving forward kept you from falling.

As children, we can learn to trust in this movement. But some may hold on, fear letting go of the bar behind them, and become immobilized. When we stop moving ahead, we get stuck or we fall. Some of us begin again; some of us, frustrated by our lack of progress, may choose to avoid and not return to the activity. Opportunities for change and growth cease.

You are the one in motion now. You have to let go of the bar behind as you move forward. There is a moment when you are holding on to nothing. And you don't fall. Your momentum—your forward motion—moves you to the next bar. This is the transformational process, the experience of transition and change. We are here to encourage you to grab the next bar and then swing ahead to the next.

Your interest in knowing more about your sexual self, however tentative, is the surest sign that you are ready to move toward an honest exploration of your feelings. Trust in your forward motion to carry you through, and savor that moment of transition.

In the next few chapters, we will be exploring some elements of early recovery. These include the following:

- **You will reflect on the effects of socialization in your life.** What impacts do the beliefs and assumptions around you have on you? What does your social environment teach you to feel about yourself?

- **You will endeavor to make some peace with your body,** just as it is, at least for now. Part of being sexual is what you do with your body. If you are uncomfortable or unfamiliar with your body, your sexuality will be affected. This does not mean you cannot experience deep connection or pleasure while also feeling insecure, living with dysmorphia (preoccupied with self-perceived defects), or experiencing gender dysphoria (distress associated with incongruence between sex assigned at birth and gender identity). It means that even if you intend to make changes to your body, you offer your body care and acceptance along the journey.

- **You will be learning about your genitals.** How important is genital stimulation to your sexual self? Do you like your genitals, fear them, feel intimidated by them, feel confused about them, feel proud of them, or try not to think about them?

- **You will enter a practice of self-pleasure.** Yes, this can include masturbation, but it encompasses so much more. A practice of self-pleasure can stand alone, or it can be a step in your journey toward deeper intimacy with others.

When you are able to give loving touch to yourself, you are more able to accept it from a partner and to know what you want from a partner.

- **You will become aware of your sexual feelings,** which exist separately from your partner or from anyone else. Your erotic life and sexual energy exist in their own right.

Try to connect with the feelings these goals stir up in you. You may feel afraid of exploring your feelings about sexuality, especially if you have been disconnected from them over time. Identifying and connecting with your feelings requires a great deal of courage. Sometimes our capacity for sexual desire and arousal recedes due to medications, menopause, injury, stress, or any number of other issues that arise in life and in recovery. We will practice attending to sensual pleasure that does not demand sexual response and go from there.

You do not have to eliminate your fear in order to be honest about your sexual feelings. Courage is acting honestly in spite of fear, knowing that the rewards of authentic self-knowledge will carry you forward on your journey of change. These rewards have a rhythm and momentum all their own—all your own.

So take courage. Please treat yourself with gentleness and patience, and allow yourself to move at your own pace.

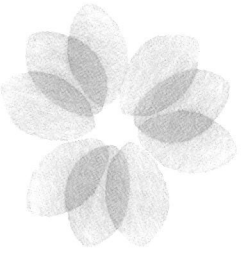

CHAPTER 1

The Past in the Present

Women totally, definitely, have been shamed and oppressed out of connecting with our real sexual selves.

———

Emily Nagoski, "My Lying Vagina, and the Lying Liars Who Lie About Her"

What does it mean to become a sexual person in our society? What does it mean to have this complex thing called sexuality integrated into our lives in a meaningful way? What is your own unique experience of pleasure, and how do you cultivate it in a way that makes you feel glad to be alive?

These are big questions. They are made even more difficult because we almost never ask them, let alone find answers for them. Our intention is to help you learn how to answer these questions for yourself.

In our work, we have been touched by the depth of pain that many women and nonbinary people feel about their sexuality. Sometimes we have become overwhelmed with grief, given the difficulties so many of us face due to violence, addiction, and the effects of childhood traumas. Overall, though, we are hopeful. Our hope comes from our own recovery and self-discovery, and then years of supporting hundreds of people to grow in self-understanding and self-love—in recovery groups, in treatment programs, in sex education classes, and in individual therapy and coaching. Experience has taught us that it is possible for you to face what is unknown or painful about your own sexuality and grow into a new, loving relationship with this part of yourself.

Our Sexual Self-Image

The subject of sexuality usually produces a paradoxical reaction: We are eager to know, but we are afraid of what we might find out. How did we come to such a confused state about something that is so basic to human existence?

Our present sexual feelings and actions do not exist in a vacuum. They are molded and influenced by everything that has happened to us in the past. By working with our past and honestly naming all that has happened to us—our gender socialization within our family, our childhood experiences, our adolescent sexual experiences, our choice of partners, our sexual behavior prior to the decision to recover—we can move into a new level of sexual freedom and expansion. When this happens, our sexual feelings and actions will arise from the present moment, not from the mixed messages, pain, confusion, or dissociation we had in the past.

Our sexual self-image begins to be formed by the messages we receive as children about gender and bodies in our home: what it means to be a man or a woman, and whether our family honors nonbinary, transgender, and gender-expansive expression. We receive both explicit, or spoken, messages and implicit, or unspoken, messages. For example, many children have experienced an affinity for a game, toy, or color, and then been told they weren't allowed to enjoy their preference because "that's not for you, it's for boys/girls." That is an explicit message about appropriate gender behavior. An implicit message occurs when women at a family gathering all begin cleaning up after a meal, while the men of the family relax and catch up in another room.

After training in the rules of gender at home, children do eventually learn about sexuality and sex itself. If your parents or caregivers seemed confused, ashamed, or embarrassed to discuss sex or even to think about it, your sexual identity was affected. You had to seek answers elsewhere—from other children or teens, secret stashes of pornography, movies, the internet. In this you are not alone. You are also not alone if you learned about sex through confusing or traumatic experiences with an older child or adult who should have been caring for you.

Even people who were offered mature, loving examples of sexuality in their homes as children may struggle to explore their own sexuality as adults because of how confusing the cultural messages are outside their home. In other words, no matter how you grew up, you have likely been affected by what author Dr. Emily Nagoski calls the "cultural lies" about sex. These lies have emerged from years of research on sexuality that acknowledged only a male/female gender binary, presumed women were the same as men, or presented women's differences as deficiencies. There are also cultural lies of omission and silence, in which victims of childhood sexual trauma are taught to feel ashamed and keep their stories to themselves.

At the same time, everybody is expected to be good at sex, though ironically it's the one activity we're not supposed to have seen anyone else do in person. Learning to be "good" at sex by watching pornography doesn't work for most people, mostly because porn is designed to be entertaining and titillating, not educational.

For most of us, adolescence brings intense and confusing physical and emotional changes that then get all mixed up with images and messages from the external world. As a result, most of us are convinced that we're not doing it "right," that others know a secret we don't possess, that we're doing it too much or too little, that we're "good" at it or "bad" at it, or that we know how or don't know how to please a partner. We're supposed to be competent and to like sex, but we're not supposed to know anything about it. It's a dirty thing we are not supposed to talk about, yet we're supposed to save it for the one we love. No wonder we're confused!

The truth is that although we are born with genitalia and the capacity for pleasure, we have to learn how to identify and express our own sexuality. For most of us—especially those of us who have used drugs or alcohol to anesthetize ourselves—this means starting by unlearning much of what we've learned about sexuality.

We can begin to untangle our mixed messages by sharing our experiences. Most of us still struggle to speak calmly about sex, what really happens, and how it feels. Increasing our ability to talk about sex in an authentic way is vital to our sexual recovery. When we can't talk about sex, when we have to keep our sexual feelings, thoughts, and experiences secret, then we are more likely to feel ashamed of them. As long as we feel ashamed, we will feel that there's something wrong with us, and we will be blocked. Our growth will necessarily be limited. It is only when we take our fragmented sexual selves out of that hidden, silent, secret place and sift through the pieces that we begin to realize the possibility of integration and expansion. This too is a potential we are born with, one we can all truly possess.

Authentic Sex Talk

When we are able to talk with someone we trust about sexuality, something wonderful happens: What we previously thought of as individual pathology—that is, what was wrong with only us or our own family—gets put into a larger context. We see that we are doing and feeling what many others are raised to do and feel. We begin to see the limitations of the provisions that our society offers women. We come to have compassion for ourselves.

We have made difficult choices while living in a social climate designed to make it nearly impossible to feel good about ourselves without clear intention and good support.

In our experience, one effective way to move through a process of sexual recovery is in a group, especially one for women, non-binary people, and gender-expansive participants. Some groups are peer led, meaning people with similar experiences share with each other and give each other support and feedback. Some groups are facilitated by a therapist, coach, or other qualified leader. Some are in person, others online. You can begin by doing a few searches for recovery groups in your area, if you are not already going to one. You should always feel free to try another, change your mind, and seek the right fit.

Groups can be very powerful, but they are certainly not the only way to begin speaking authentically about our sexuality. You may choose to share your feelings with a friend, in individual therapy with a professional counselor, via sexuality coaching, with a trusted partner, or in a workbook or journal.

This book will give you the opportunity to hear a variety of women discuss their sexual history and recovery. We hope you find that one or more of their threads interweaves with yours. We also hope that you see how others' experiences, different from your own, can contribute to your understanding of yourself and your wider community. Here are a few people whose voices you will hear throughout this book.

Michelle: Keeping It All Together

Michelle is thirty-nine, with wavy brown hair that swirls below her shoulders and an understated, natural makeup look. She is a cheerful, organized, white, middle-class, heterosexual, married mother of two. Michelle keeps a sharp eye on herself in the mirror, monitoring for new wrinkles, "extra" pounds, and gray hairs.

Michelle's mother managed to keep a household together while Michelle's father drank before, during, and after work for decades. Because he wasn't physically violent, and their material needs and wants were met, Michelle has always considered herself lucky and her childhood in an alcoholic family "not that bad."

A few years before she got married to Chris, Michelle was sexually assaulted by a co-worker at the firm where she worked as a paralegal. She filed a complaint with her human resources department, but there were no consequences. This discouraged her from filing a police report. While the experience terrified her, she told only one girlfriend at the time, worried that others in the office might see her as deserving of the assault. She thought they might think she seduced the co-worker because he had shown interest in her over several months. Her friend helped her quit and find a new job. Michelle still does her best never to be alone in a room with a man who isn't her husband. "There's no reason to risk it," she says with a shrug.

Michelle fell in love with Chris, a software developer, and they married and had their first child within a year, and their second two years later. Both children were healthy, and Michelle's mother and sister helped out when the babies were very small. When COVID-19 hit and Michelle and Chris had to stay home with their two young children, she realized she enjoyed it more than working in an office. Because Chris was making more money than he had before, they decided Michelle could be a stay-at-home parent until both of their children were in grade school.

Once Chris returned to the office, however, Michelle found stay-at-home parenting much more stressful. She started taking a daily prescription for anxiety. Her habit of drinking a glass of wine at night grew to two, three, often a whole bottle, or more. She and her friends would joke about becoming #winemoms, and

Michelle began adding a fast-acting anti-anxiety medication and a sleeping pill to her nightly routine, prescribed by her primary care doctor. She told her doctor she drank one to three drinks per week.

Michelle is proud of her beautiful home and her happy, healthy children, and she knows her life looks great from the outside. Most Sundays, Michelle goes out to "boozy brunch" with her friends and usually comes home drunk. Regularly, she is blacked out and sick for hours those evenings.

Recently, when Michelle had a particularly unpleasant hangover after a brunch, Chris gave her the silent treatment for a few days. She finally goaded him into talking with her, and he got uncharacteristically angry. He told Michelle she was turning out just like her father and that he was sick of it. Michelle was hurt, angry, and defensive. She considered her drinking to be under control—she rarely drank before putting her kids in the car, which her father had done regularly. She didn't drink first thing in the morning, and there were days here and there when she didn't drink much. She focused on how angry Chris had become and told him he was being controlling.

Now Michelle and Chris have an isolating nighttime routine of screen time in separate rooms before falling asleep. She doesn't want to count the weeks or months it has been since they connected sexually. Michelle feels ashamed to admit it, but her fear of rejection and her defensiveness are so strong she doesn't dare approach Chris, even for nonsexual, affectionate touch. Without Chris initiating, Michelle feels trapped in a cycle of wanting to connect but feeling a chasm between them that she doesn't know how to cross. At the same time, she is not masturbating or enjoying her body in any other way.

Michelle continues to use alcohol and prescription medication to calm her anxiety every night, and she has started shopping more too—she goes online and clicks on ads for clothing and household items, which she tells Chris are "for the kids," "to help the house," or "because I needed it." They are no longer able to pay off their credit cards every month, but Michelle can't stop ordering, and packages keep coming. She tells her doctor she needs more pills, but her doctor expresses concern at how many she is already taking and says she can't have any more fast-acting anxiety medication before next month's refill. This leads Michelle to drink even more, late at night after everyone is asleep.

On the outside, their family still seems perfect, but on the inside, Michelle is struggling to keep it all together. She suggests couple's therapy, hoping they can repair their relationship before things get any worse. Chris agrees to go. Michelle tells a good friend she is ready to try something new in her marriage, but she has not told anyone about the conflict they have about her drinking, use of prescription pills, and spending.

Nova: Sobriety Just Isn't Sexy

Nova's parents were adventurers who met at the Burning Man festival in the late 1990s and spent the ensuing months together, following their favorite bands on tour, until Nova's mother was too far along in her pregnancy to camp in a tent comfortably. Nova's young, idealistic parents joined an intentional spiritual community, where Nova was born. Nova's father was from Mexico and had migrated to the United States with his family as a boy. Nova's mother, a white self-proclaimed hippie from a small New England town, eventually left the spiritual community and gave Nova's father full custody. Nova says of her mother, "I love her as a friend. But she didn't raise me, so I call her 'Mom' mostly as a courtesy." Nova was raised in a nontraditional household of nearly twenty people.

Nova had very little contact with mainstream society until she was a teenager because the intentional community was self-sufficient and homeschooled the children. She was taught about her body, sex, and procreation without shame, and she was comfortable in sexual exploration as a teenager with both boys and girls.

When the community dissolved and Nova had to enter a public high school, she was shocked at how the students treated each other. "It was the first time anyone made me feel like my brown skin was a big problem," she recalls. She was not accepted by other students and found herself spending a lot of time alone or with one or two other "weirdos." She kept passing grades, but she had to work to support herself. Her father was not home most of the time because he did seasonal work and traveled on his off time.

Now, at twenty-five, Nova knows more about living in the "default" world. After graduating high school, she spent nearly two years in what she now calls "a kind of limbo." She had difficulty conforming to the demands of low-paying jobs and struggled to find stable housing and pay basic bills. When Nova was nineteen, her roommate brought her to an audition at a strip club, and she has been working there as a dancer for six years.

Nova learned how to do challenging pole tricks and quickly gained status in the club. She takes great joy in her body and its capacities, and she has a large following on social media who respond to her beauty, her reflections on life and spirituality, and her bubbly personality. The flexible schedule allows Nova freedom to pursue her creative interests and build more social connections.

Nova says she felt "a lot of pressure to party with customers" in her early days and developed some destructive habits to cope. Many nights, she would drink at pace with the men she was entertaining, black out, and either wake up at home without knowing how she got there or, worse, with someone she hadn't consciously consented to have sex with. Nova followed the advice of another dancer at her club and added uppers to the mix, relying on cocaine and methamphetamine to stop the blackouts.

She felt physically safer staying awake, but she also became increasingly paranoid, withdrawn, and preoccupied with managing hangovers and comedowns and hiding her drug use from prying eyes. Because thinness was so valued at the club, Nova was initially told she looked great, even when her weight loss was a symptom of active addiction. After three years on that roller coaster, Nova remembers, "Another girl at the club literally put her finger in my face and told me to get sober." Nova adds, "I knew she was right. I went with her to a meeting." While Alcoholics Anonymous was her entry point to recovery, Nova felt excluded by the language and some of the ideas. She asked her friend if there was anything else. "Start something," her friend told her.

Once she had made it through the difficult first weeks of withdrawal, Nova founded an online sober community meeting for women who worked in the adult industries: sex workers, strip club performers, webcam models, and porn performers who needed an alternative to traditional recovery. They met once a week and offered each other peer support. Luckily for Nova, a few of the members had been through methamphetamine addiction withdrawal and were able to give her good advice for managing her cravings.

At the club, Nova created friendships with other sober or sober-curious dancers, and she enlisted the help of the bartenders to make her mocktails while she was entertaining customers. She slowly learned how to create better boundaries with customers. She read recovery literature, practiced daily meditations, and started feeling healthier. Now, younger dancers turn to Nova for advice and support.

One consequence of sobriety Nova hadn't expected was that she was no longer dating or creating space for sexual connection in her personal life. "I used to feel pretty relaxed about sex," she says, "but I got used to drinking and being high to make it happen. I want that confidence I had when I was a kid, but I don't know how to get there. I know how to act sexy; I do it for a living! But deep down I don't *feel* that sexy within myself. It's a performance for customers. I'm not sure who I am sexually, or what I want, or if I even have real sexual feelings of my own."

Tamara: Back to Square One

Tamara is a tenured professor of history and African American studies at a large university, where she has won numerous teaching awards. Early in her career, she published her dissertation with an academic press, and it still is used in history courses at various campuses. She often speaks publicly about her experiences of tokenism and misogynoir (the combined force of anti-Black racism and misogyny directed toward Black women) at conferences for women in academia. Between writing, teaching, mentoring students, serving on committees, and speaking at conferences, Tamara's work occupies most of her time and attention.

At sixty-three, Tamara is reluctantly single again, after a difficult divorce from her wife. Tamara's elderly mother, Anne, has moved into Tamara's small house in an effort to cut costs because of Anne's increasing need for caregiving. Anne is a devout Christian who has never been comfortable with Tamara's sexual orientation, even though she was always kind and respectful to Alisha, Tamara's ex-wife. Anne and Tamara live amicably, but Tamara is always aware of her mother's disapproval.

"I love Mom, but I am smaller in spirit around her," Tamara tells her therapist. "She would be so happy if I would just break down and find a good man. She still talks like that's possible. I'm so tired."

Years ago, Tamara had a serious car accident and was prescribed an opioid pain medication while she recovered from a series of back surgeries. She still has chronic pain and takes a combination of prescription opioids, over-the-counter ibuprofen, and an anti-convulsant for nerve pain. Some days, she needs a cane to walk around campus.

For years, her medication has dulled the terrible pain from her injuries, but it has also contributed to her feeling more and more disconnected from her body. Menopause didn't help, either, as Tamara lost all interest in sex, which hurt Alisha and contributed to the issues in their marriage. Before the accident, Tamara remembers feeling more joy in her body. "It used to be, you invite me to your wedding," she says, "and I'm on the dance floor until they cut the lights."

In therapy, Tamara is talking about grieving: her divorce, her increasing physical pain, her mother's signs of aging. She is afraid of getting older without a companion, but she also feels totally overwhelmed by the prospect of dating someone new. ("What am I supposed to do, go to the bar and then bring a woman home to meet Mom?") Tamara did not date many women before she met Alisha, and she feels like an outsider, even among her lesbian friends.

Tamara can name all of the issues she's facing, but she is frustrated by a sense that there is nothing she can do to change her situation. When asked what she wants, she is quick to answer "love and companionship," but then she says she feels like she'd have to cross an impossible distance to get it.

After six months in therapy focused on the daily struggles of her work, back pain, adjusting to living with her mother, and dealing with the fallout from her divorce, there was a crisis at home. Anne went to the bathroom, took a serious fall, and couldn't get up off the floor. She called out but was unable to wake Tamara. Anne stayed stuck in a painful position for hours with a fractured hip. When Tamara finally woke up from her deep, medicated sleep and was able to help, Anne was in terrible pain, had urinated in her clothing, and needed an ambulance.

In therapy, Tamara divulges that she has needed to get "extra" painkillers, bought from a student, to manage her pain. She had accepted the fact of physical dependence after a doctor told her she would live the rest of her life taking narcotics for her back pain. However, she had always taken the pills as prescribed until last year. Something has changed. She is sure that if she hadn't been so heavily medicated that night, she would have been able to help her mother right away. Instead, she was passed out. Tamara feels afraid, ashamed, alone, and out of control.

Ash: Adversity, Recovery, Relapse, Repeat

Ash is a thirty-three-year-old peer recovery specialist at a small treatment center. Ash came out as nonbinary and started using they/them pronouns during their first stay in a rehabilitation facility more than seven years ago. Because of relapse, Ash counts three years sober, but their recovery story began long before they entered rehab for the first time.

Ash was sexually abused by their stepfather from age four until ten, when they told a teacher at school what was happening. Ash was removed from their home. Ash's mother was addicted to heroin and was not able to create a safe home for Ash to return to. Ash remembers their mother giving them their first cigarette and sip of beer when Ash was six years old.

Ash bounced from one foster care home to another, eventually spending two years in a girls' group home until they turned eighteen. At the home, Ash had a sexual relationship with a male staff member, who gave them more freedoms than the other girls. "I wasn't popular," Ash remembers. "But I never felt like I fit in with the girls anyway, so I didn't care."

"I did feel guilty about my little sisters," Ash says, "because they were still living with that monster, and I couldn't protect them." When Ash's mother died, Ash's sisters went into foster care as well, and Ash is no longer in contact with them.

Ash describes themself as a "garbage head," meaning they would take any drug offered to them, although they consistently used alcohol and heroin throughout their late teens and twenties. "It's not just that I'll replace one drug with another," Ash tells their peer group, "it's that I'll take any of them, anytime."

Ash describes living with a small group of other young people who were using drugs. They would take turns getting high in an extended-stay motel room, and most of them were involved in street-based sex work and drug trades. "I was the only one trying to keep a legit job," Ash remembers, "because I had my ID and references from the group home. But I couldn't keep any of those jobs, even if I was fucking the manager." Ash remembers that during this time they had "a lot of sex I didn't really want to have, but it got me something I needed."

Eventually, Ash was arrested for driving under the influence and without a license. Because they couldn't pay the fines, they spent three months in jail. That was the first time they thought recovery might be a possibility, because "AA meetings were one of the only things we got to do." Once released from jail, they spent some time doing inpatient rehab. It was there that Ash found the courage to come out as nonbinary. Later, Ash was able to stay with a friend who didn't struggle with addiction, and Ash kept going to meetings.

"I never told my sponsor anything about the abuse," Ash recalls. "So when we hit the Fourth Step, and I started panicking, she didn't understand." The Fourth Step asks a participant to make "a searching and fearless moral inventory of ourselves." Most traditional Twelve Step programs require people to take a specific look at their sexual conduct and take responsibility for harms they may have caused.

Like many who have been victimized sexually, Ash found this process triggering, and they quit attending meetings during their Fourth Step process. They felt they had gotten all they needed out of the program and were on the right track, and they were able to maintain sobriety on their own, for a time.

Three years ago, Ash was in a healthier relationship than they'd ever had before but was still struggling with panic attacks and nightmares. When the daily stress of life got to be too much, Ash's behavior became erratic. At first only Ben, their partner, noticed the difference, but eventually it became undeniable.

Ash showed up to their partner Ben's workplace unexpectedly, crying uncontrollably. They were convinced that they were being stalked and followed, but Ben didn't see anyone matching the description Ash gave. One night, Ben became afraid. Ash was screaming, threatening to use a gun on themselves or Ben, and so Ben called the police.

Ash was hospitalized on an involuntary seventy-two-hour psychiatric hold, given powerful antipsychotic and mood-stabilizing medications, and released without a plan for continued care. Their part-time job did not offer health insurance, and no one called to follow up with Ash.

Within a month, they were experiencing withdrawal from the medications and sought relief in familiar substances. Ben set a boundary and ended the relationship, asking Ash to move out.

Ash spent a week living out of their car, staying high as much as possible, before "something snapped inside. I wasn't mad at Ben; I was mad at my stepdad. I let myself cry and scream for a while. Then I walked to a church in town that I knew had Alcoholics Anonymous meetings at night and sat outside until they opened the doors."

After three years of sobriety this time around, and with clients at the treatment center where they work looking up to them, Ash is determined to stay in recovery. "I know I have to take a look at my childhood in a new way," they say. "There's a box of feelings I locked up a long time ago. I thought I had to keep them locked up, or I might die. But locking them up was killing me too." Sexual recovery scares Ash, but they know it is an important part of the journey ahead.

Discovering Our Sexual Selves

Michelle, Nova, Tamara, and Ash are struggling with their unique experiences and the tangled messages they received, both from their families' legacies and from society while growing up. They all received messages about their worth as human beings, and how their gender and sexuality affected their worth. For each, there is a journey ahead.

Michelle learned early that physical appearance is important, but she received confusing messages about sexuality: that it's important to be concerned about how your body looks, but only one man, your husband, should notice it, and he should decide when and how sex happens. Consciously, Michelle would not want to replicate the alcoholism from her own family of origin, and she certainly feels more sexually aware than her mother seemed to be. However, Michelle is trapped, trying to live up to enormous unspoken expectations of being a good wife and mother while denying the impact of her past traumatic experiences. So, she is managing her own stress and anxiety with alcohol and pills. Michelle's unconscious solution has been to disconnect from herself and her sexuality through substances that dull her body's responses and repress the cumulative pain of her fragmented experiences.

Unlike Michelle, who was raised to be critical of her own body, Nova was socialized to be sexually confident and egalitarian with her peers in the intentional community where she grew up. Her father and the other adults there tried hard to raise Nova in a permissive atmosphere that encouraged exploration and openness. Because of this, Nova is at ease with physical sexuality. However, she has found that a personal connection with her own desires, wants, needs, and fantasies is missing. She is graceful and expert at creating memorable erotic experiences for customers, and she is a good friend and mentor in her community, but recovery has revealed a space where she needs self-awareness. She is beginning to recognize this and would like to reconnect her emotional life with her body and sexual activity.

Tamara grew up without words to identify her feelings and experiences, and she always felt like an outsider in her anti-gay, Christian family. Still, she maintains a deep love for her mother, who is now living with her and experiencing a new level of physical dependence as she ages. Working with a years-old disability herself, Tamara has accomplished a great deal in her career despite the racism, sexism, and ableism in her workplace. Still grieving her divorce, and not completely sure why her marriage ended, she struggles to feel deep, adult, human connection, and she has given up on hoping for a return to sexual pleasure.

When Ash got sober the first time, they were able to connect with a more authentic gender identity inside, and they had the courage and support to come out as nonbinary. Through a series of relapses and increasing consequences for their alcohol and drug use, Ash has come to understand that their childhood sexual trauma does need more healing attention for their recovery to progress. Ash is resourceful, caring, and self-reflective. However, they can also be impulsive and self-harming. The mental health consequences of their childhood experiences have had far-reaching effects in their life, and Ash seeks to create more healthy habits and patterns.

Understanding our gender identity—whether it is clear and fixed (as it is for many cisgender women), different from what we were taught as children, fluid, expansive, or changing—is a process that can happen simultaneously with the work of understanding our sexuality. Even for those who feel very clear about their gender, there is great value in taking a look at the socialization we receive, beginning the moment someone decides "it's a girl!" or "it's a boy!" Gender and sexuality interact and affect each other, and your experience of your gender is a welcome part of discovering your sexual self.

The message implicit in all the experiences you will encounter in this book is that sexuality is much more than sexual behavior. Sexuality can be a lifelong process of discovery, an important part of who we are and how we are in the world, regardless of how much desire we do or don't feel and whether we have a partner. As you move with these and other women and gender-expansive people on their personal journeys of sexual recovery, we hope you will begin to become aware of the components of your own sexuality: its complexity, its history, and its uniqueness. These are your legacies to claim and explore.

○ ○ ○

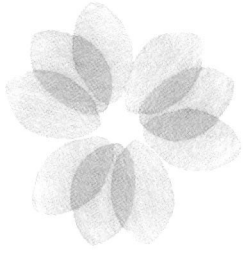

CHAPTER 2

Inauthenticity and Contradictions

We have had the truth of our bodies withheld from us or distorted; we have been kept in ignorance of our most intimate places. Our instincts have been punished . . . it has been difficult, too, to know the lies of our complicity from the lies we believed.

———

Adrienne Rich, *On Lies, Secrets, and Silence: Selected Prose 1966–1978*

Sexual inauthenticity comes in many guises. You may pretend not to understand a joke. You may claim to have had fewer partners than you have. You may "forget" to bring barrier protection (condoms, diaphragm, dental dams) on a date, even though you have every intention of having sex. You may get drunk, knowing you are more likely to initiate or allow sex that way. You may fake an orgasm to please your lover. You may continue to participate in a sex act even when you'd rather not. Performance to please someone else: That's what it's often about.

Our participation in sex we don't prefer isn't necessarily the core problem. Sometimes, we have sex to stay safe in the moment with a person we can't fully trust to be kind if we say no. Sometimes, a sexual performance is part of how we make our living, like Nova's job dancing in a strip club. Sometimes, we try something new with a partner who asks us to, and we don't love it. Having sexual experiences we don't prefer can be a valuable tool for our survival or self-knowledge. What matters in recovery is how conscious we are of our participation in sex we don't prefer, why we are doing it, and taking stock of how it affects us.

Sometimes we get so lost in being sexual the way our partner wants us to, or the way we were taught we should, or the way we've seen in movies or shows, or the only way we know how, that we aren't able to sense what brings us our own true pleasure. When we perform sexually for others more than we authentically engage with our body's likes and dislikes, we can get lost and out of balance.

This is not to say that being generous with our partners is a problem—on the contrary. *Referred pleasure,* or the joy we feel when our partner is experiencing their own pleasure, is a real thing. Attentiveness, generosity, and joy at being a "giver" are lovely expressions of sexuality when they are freely offered and felt.

What we seek is self-awareness, so we can be fully at choice whenever we are sexual. In this chapter, we will explore the ways we have been taught to live in denial of our sexuality and begin to reconnect honestly with our own sources of pleasure.

Many people who have experienced trauma or addiction have become so distanced from their sexuality that they despair of ever being able to bring their inner and outer sexual selves into harmony. This was co-author Stephanie's experience. Being in recovery for alcoholism affected her sexuality as much as it affected the other aspects of her being. It was only when she became sober that she began to realize the degree to which her alcoholism had anesthetized and distorted her sexuality.

Stephanie started drinking in college, where heavy drinking just seemed normal. This continued through her graduate program and into her married life. Stephanie's active sex life before and during marriage was almost always combined with alcohol, and all of her sexual experience was with men. Stephanie was curious about sex starting in childhood, but sex was never spoken of at home, in high school, or in college. Today she finds this a little surprising, given that she grew up during the sexual revolution and the women's movements of the 1960s and 1970s! Regardless, she followed expectations until her drinking made life unmanageable. In her mid-thirties, Stephanie finally acknowledged that alcohol was a problem.

The saddest part was that during her early recovery no one told her that she would need to explore her sexuality. No one pointed to the sexual problems that she might encounter in sobriety, and no one reassured her that many women had similar experiences. In her first year of recovery, Stephanie divorced, left the East Coast, and moved back to California, where she was from.

When Stephanie was drinking, she was attracted to women, but she thought it was just the alcohol. Once she was sober and still feeling attracted to women, she knew she needed to address it. During her first year in a PhD program, Stephanie met and dated a woman for the first time. Now she jokes, "It was drinking that allowed me to stay married and heterosexual." Once sober, she had to face how much of her own sexual feeling she had hidden from herself.

Denial of sexual concerns often extends to therapists, recovery counselors, and Twelve Step groups. Unless a therapist has received specialized training for sex therapy, or the group is dedicated to sexual and relationship concerns, conversations about sexuality are often awkward and uncomfortable. Yet, as we know, only when denial is examined and replaced with truth and understanding does change become possible. We become whole by making our behavior consistent with our feelings as much as we safely can.

The recovery process demands that we become familiar with our inner lives and that we express our inner selves authentically in the world. If we are unable to see the relationship between our thoughts, feelings, beliefs, and interactions with others, and stay consistent on all these levels, we will be unable to live our lives with meaning and fulfillment. We have to be honest with ourselves first.

Unfortunately, the external world is also a place of inauthenticity and contradiction when it comes to sexuality. America's moralistic attitude toward sexuality is so deeply ingrained that it is often invisible. We live in a patriarchal society in which heterosexual women's and LGBTQ+ people's sexual desires and expression have been systematically attacked or diminished. Sexual behavior is simultaneously inaccurately represented in most mainstream media. We may be surrounded by sexualized imagery, but our access to comprehensive sex education in schools has been on the decline since the 1990s.

At the same time, there has been a proliferation of private sex education trying to bridge the gaps. You can find sex educators creating podcasts, making social media content, running YouTube channels, selling private courses, and hosting conferences. Many of them are highly trained and skilled. The barrier is usually that you must search them out on your own. If you know already that you haven't had access to comprehensive sex education, check the Resources section at the end of the book for some suggestions on where to begin.

In other words, most of us have not had consistent access to the tools and information we need to explore our sexuality safely. Beginning from that understanding helps us to see why so many of us learn to close our hearts, minds, and bodies to our sexual feelings, or to feel ashamed and alone when we act on them. We function today as products of our history and the complex present moment.

Silencing the Inner Voice

When Michelle and Chris arrived at their first couple's therapy appointment, Michelle felt awful: nervous, scared, angry, and defensive. Chris seemed withdrawn, and his silence exacerbated her discomfort. They drove without talking and walked single file into the waiting room. Once they were seated on the couch in the therapist's office, Michelle was surprised when the therapist opened with a question about what was working well in their marriage. Chris looked at her, and she saw how sad he seemed.

They were able to list some of the more functional aspects of their partnership: They both loved their kids, they kept a beautiful home, they had a vacation planned for later in the year. Then the therapist asked about their "intimacy," which they both took to be a euphemism for their sex life. Michelle was instantly embarrassed and uncomfortable. She had talked with her girlfriends about her sex life with Chris in the early days, but this therapist was a stranger.

When she began to think about her sexual relationship with Chris, she couldn't stay thinking about it. Her attention went somewhere—anywhere—else. She looked at the curtains behind the therapist, then at the intricate pattern on the rug. Chris finally spoke up. "We haven't had a lot of intimacy," he said flatly. "With the kids and everything else . . ." he trailed off. What was he trying to say? The therapist waited for him to finish his thought, but he just shrugged.

The therapist explained that she defined *intimacy* as anything that made them feel close, connected, and on the same team. It didn't have to be sex, although that was important to many couples. She asked Michelle what helped her feel connected with Chris. "I don't know," Michelle said. She searched for something else to say, but she couldn't come up with anything substantial.

Sensing that talking about intimacy was going to be difficult, the therapist helped them navigate a beginning conversation about how mutual enjoyment, like moments of laughter and appreciation of each other, had happened for them until now. Chris answered most of the questions, while Michelle nodded and watched his face and hands move.

Neither Michelle nor Chris brought up the fight that started their current stalemate. The therapist didn't ask about substance use in their history and focused on practical ways the two of them could initiate more connection in daily life. She suggested that every day, for ten minutes, they make an effort to talk to each other about something other than work, children, the house, or their relationship.

Michelle had trouble listening, and when they left the appointment, she felt bewildered and couldn't remember what had happened in the therapist's office. Chris seemed more cheerful, though, so she agreed to go to back in two weeks.

Being honest, especially with ourselves, is a necessary first step toward changing our patterns. The difficulty concentrating that Michelle experienced in the therapist's office, and the way she immediately forgot what happened, add up to a form of self-protection many survivors of trauma will recognize. It is called *dissociation*. When asked to face the difficult feelings she was going through and share vulnerability with Chris, Michelle's system shut down. She wasn't consciously choosing this. Dissociation is a sign that we are overwhelmed and need to slow down, back up, and receive more support.

In Michelle's case, dissociation happened in part because she hadn't yet been honest with herself about her own feelings and her own behavior. For some people, honesty comes as a private revelation. For others, it feels safer to be with another person when big feelings are ready to come out. This can change over time too. Perfect conditions rarely exist, so it is up to each recovering person to seek their own true feelings in the ways that are safest for them. Michelle has yet to do this.

Another piece of the puzzle is that Michelle was socialized to embrace unspoken ideals about romantic relationships and sex. She always assumed she would marry a great man and have enjoyable sex with him for the rest of her life. She would never speak this aloud—it would sound a little silly, even to her. However, it had never occurred to her that falling in love and getting married was only the beginning of a sexual relationship.

Michelle has not considered that her experience as the child of a person with an addiction to alcohol, or her experience of sexual assault, may affect her capacity for intimacy years later. She was not prepared for the difficulties of maintaining a sexual relationship after having children or during a stressful event like the COVID-19 lockdowns. Sex stopped being a priority for her once her trauma symptoms and self-medication took over. For Michelle, talking about sex and intimate feelings is terribly scary, like opening Pandora's box, and she isn't ready to even peek inside yet.

In families where shame drives a large amount of everyone's behavior, such as families with addiction, abuse, or other painful issues, it is common to see something called a "no-talk rule." A no-talk rule can apply to anything that would disrupt the status quo. For example, children do not talk about a parent's addiction, parents do not talk about a partner's infidelity, no one talks about the abuse happening in the family, and so on.

The no-talk rule is also a familiar fixture in most of our sexual lives. This rule has a variety of forms, such as: It's not okay to talk about sex, even to ask for what you want. If your partner really loved you, you would get just what you wanted and needed in bed. When the right person comes along, it's going to be perfect. If it's not perfect, there must be something wrong with you, your body, or your technique. If it was easy at first, but something has changed, there is something wrong with you—better avoid bringing it up. And on and on.

Even for people who have addressed some of the no-talk rules that mainstream culture hands us about sex, there are usually some others lurking in the background. Maybe a polyamorous community has a no-talk rule about the self-destructive behavior of a beloved partner. Perhaps a couple is okay with their current sex life but has a no-talk rule about introducing anything deemed kinky, even though one partner fantasizes about kink nonstop.

These rules can prohibit us from ending an unsatisfactory relationship, from asking for what we want, and from taking responsibility for our own sexuality. A no-talk rule from child-hood trains us to shut up and ignore uncomfortable truths, and dissociation is one way we may continue this habit. The only way to know if we are abiding by these rules is to create increasing honesty within ourselves.

Sex as a Means to an End

As a child enduring sexual abuse, Ash learned that if they lay still and quiet, the terrible moment would end quicker, and afterward their stepfather would treat them very nicely for a day or two. Unconsciously, this lesson stuck. As a teenager, Ash tried to take control of their situation by creating relationships with people who had power over their life: sleeping with a staff member at their group home to gain more freedoms and having sex with a manager at their job to smooth over problems they'd created while they were high. Ash had sex in exchange for drugs, a place to sleep, a meal, anything that would help them survive to the next day and the next opportunity to get high. Ash learned early that sex could get them something they wanted or needed. Sex they didn't want seemed like a small price to pay for survival.

While working their first Twelve Step program, Ash focused exclusively on getting sober. Importantly, Alcoholics Anonymous and most Twelve Step groups based on it aren't designed to support victims of childhood sexual abuse. Doing a "searching and fearless moral inventory" of their own sexual history without the context of their original abuse threw Ash into a panic.

At some level, they knew they might need to make amends to people they harmed in the process of getting their own needs met while actively addicted. However, without processing the fact of their own sexual trauma, Ash risked taking on more blame and shame than was theirs to hold.

Ash felt shame about "seducing" the staff member at their group home. But that adult had been charged with Ash's care and was the one responsible. This is a set of extremely difficult experiences to untangle, and Ash did not have adequate support during their first attempt at recovery. They left their Twelve Step group without clarity on their own sexual history.

It took a series of relapses and mental health crises for Ash to finally be ready to face the pain of their early childhood abuse and begin the process of recovering their own adult sexuality. When they began unpacking their sexual history with a trauma therapist, Ash realized they had been sexually exploited many times, and it was a painful revelation.

The things we do when we are in the grip of addiction and trauma can be extremely harmful to ourselves and other people. At the time, we are utterly convinced that the ends justify the means. Part of any recovery process is taking responsibility and accountability for the harms we have caused to others. At the same time, it should make sense that people who have survived sexual trauma can have real difficulty with traditional accountability processes like the ones used by Twelve Step groups. This is due to many reasons, including the reality that survivors are often blamed directly for the abuse they survived, and sometimes the internalization of this blame becomes a long-term, totalizing sense of shame that coexists with the shame of addiction and other out-of-control behaviors.

Co-author Vanessa remembers a therapist urging them to enact better self-care while they were struggling in their mid-twenties. The therapist wanted Vanessa to focus on eating three meals a day, rather than only one (and often none), and to create some stronger boundaries inside a relationship that had slid from emotional abuse to physical violence.

Vanessa's self-worth had been eroded by multiple forces. Some were subtle and chronic, like the sexism and homophobia in their family, while others were more dramatic, like intimate partner violence and sexual trauma. For years, Vanessa agreed to unwanted sex to appease rageful partners.

When the therapist asked Vanessa to consider some new self-care practices, Vanessa recalls telling the therapist, "I just don't see why I should take better care of a self that has been such a disappointment."

"Disappointment or not," the therapist said, "this is the only self you will be issued in this life. You cannot take pride in yourself in the future if you do not begin to care for yourself now."

Vanessa did not immediately pop up off the couch and start a new life full of self-love. There were years of struggle with more trauma and out-of-control drug use before these words became truly useful and a guiding principle in their recovery. We can only hear what we need to hear when we are ready.

Physical and sexual abuse are unfortunately not uncommon experiences. These experiences affect nearly every part of us: our sense of self, our cognition, our physical health, our faith in our own perceptions, our relationships, and so on. Sexual recovery can mean facing experiences where we were not fully at choice, where we were physically unsafe, overpowered, or betrayed by someone who was supposed to care for us. Sexual recovery can mean facing a very painful history of sexual experiences we wish had not happened.

At the same time, sexual recovery can also mean facing sexual choices we would not repeat, or ways we pressured others and used them as a means to an end.

Our accountability processes need to reflect the truth of our own behavior, and at the same time, we need to be clear about the behavior of others that was *their* responsibility. If your own history still feels somewhat unclear, that is understandable. You will receive continuing support for sorting out your own responsibility and that of others in the coming chapters.

Social Lies

Social lies are the lies that our family, community, culture, and larger society teach us. All of us are affected by these myths, whether we believe them or not. Social lies become institutionalized—they are passed down from parent to child; taught in schools, religions, and legal systems; and reinforced by governmental policy and law. It is important that we become aware of the detrimental effects these lies have on our lives.

Identifying the lies can be risky—it may feel as if we reinforce their power by repeating them. On the contrary, because each of these social lies continues to have drastic consequences for women, nonbinary people, and gender-expansive people, we seek to offer you information you can use to counter them in your own life.

Lie #1: Addiction makes you a bad person.

As many of us know already, some of the decisions we made while actively involved in our addiction harmed ourselves and others, and we would not make them again. Many of us also have endured harm caused by another person who may have been struggling with their own addiction or trauma.

Co-author Stephanie has spent much of the past thirty years creating and implementing recovery programs for incarcerated women. Over and over again, she has seen women who caused harm, sometimes violence, or even loss of life, recover and find ways to rebuild their lives upon release. Stephanie estimates that nearly all of the women she has worked with who got caught up in the criminal legal system were already victims of trauma long before they got there.

Many incarcerated women were trying to protect a male partner by holding his drugs or covering for his violence. Some incarcerated women hurt their own abusers in an effort to protect their children. Thousands of women are criminalized for the consequences of their addictions. Another untold story of our prison system is how many women enter without a substance use disorder but leave with one as they attempt to self-medicate the trauma of incarceration itself.

Humans are not simply good or bad, nor are they disposable. Addiction is, for so many, a symptom of pain. As Gabor Maté says, "Don't ask why the addiction, ask why the pain."

If we can stop feeling compelled to decide who is good and who is bad, and turn our focus to the more difficult, complex question of why someone is in pain, we open ourselves to the possibility of recovery as a society. If we can turn this focus on ourselves, we open ourselves to the possibility of recovery individually. This change in mindset is truly challenging, especially for women and gender-diverse people, because of the increased stigma we endure about addiction to begin with. Because we experience more stigma than men, we sometimes have greater denial, or greater shame, about our behaviors.

Addiction has been called a disease of denial. Denial may describe some of our process—we know that addiction clouds what we see. We also know that underneath this cloud is often fear and shame. We feel fear about making change and shame about our behavior, which can turn into shame about our whole self.

This cloudiness and shame pushes us to continue in our addiction, whether it is to alcohol, drugs, or any out-of-control behavior. We can feel the distortion in our relationships as we act in violation of our values and integrity, but we can't seem to stop. This conflict increases the tension and contradictions we live in. And the cycle continues. This is when the story about being a "bad person" can begin to take hold.

Breaking out of this pattern starts with a desire and a willingness to look at things with a new awareness. Without awareness we remain trapped, unable to change and unable to see the need for change. When we are unaware of our honest thoughts, feelings, desires, and motivations, we cannot see how they relate to our behavior. They become blocked and block each other.

To move away from the protective mechanism of unawareness means to become more aware of who we are, what we feel, what we think, and why we do things. We may reconnect with our inner selves or connect for the first time; doing this gives us more understanding of why we act the way we do, and we gain integration and motivation to stay connected to our own inner self.

Sexual recovery starts with a decision to expand our consciousness, to stop using all-or-nothing terms like "bad person" for ourselves or anyone else. Recovery proceeds because of a willingness to become and to remain attentive and receptive to our true selves, which are complex, filled with good, bad, neutral, and confusing parts. Moving toward greater integrity allows our sexuality to awaken and blossom.

It takes courage to begin to strip away the layers of inauthenticity built up over the years and to look with a clear eye at our experiences, behaviors, and patterns. But acknowledging the truth and facing the pain begins a process of healing. We deserve to heal and move forward. Behavior we regret does not need to define us for the rest of our lives. And as we heal, we can begin to let our true sexual selves emerge.

Lie #2: Some bodies are better than others.

There is no denying that gender, size, race, age, and ability affect each of us in our daily lives. Each of these aspects of our lived experience (and many more, of course) opens us to greater privilege or marginalization. The consequences are vast, affect generations, and can affect every aspect of life. Some bodies are *treated as if* they are better than others, no doubt about it.

Some bodies, being treated worse than others, can feel worse to live in.

Which body would you prefer to have: one that is likely to be labeled as wrong or lacking in some way or one that is likely to be labeled as beautiful, handsome, healthy, and correct? The answer may seem obvious.

The more challenging questions are: What would change if everyone stopped seeing some bodies as better than others? What would change if everyone truly believed that all bodies were equally deserving of life, love, and care?

Everything.

Currently, women experience more issues with mental health than men do. Some people believe women are more likely to have mental health issues than men because women are more emotional. They believe it's just a sad fact that women aren't as emotionally strong as men are.

We believe women are more likely to have mental health issues because they experience higher levels of stress living in patriarchal and sexist social structures, where they are subjected to violence at higher rates than men. Women are evaluated by a medicalized mental health system that brings with it a long history of over-pathologizing women's bodies, not doing adequate research on the female body, while simultaneously dismissing women's concerns and pain.

Another example of the harms caused by the "better/worse body" belief is that right now, public misinformation about body size affects how people in larger bodies are treated socially and medically, with drastic consequences. Recent studies have shown that the long-held belief that a person with a higher body mass index (BMI) is at greater risk of a host of medical issues is a dangerous oversimplification of medical facts. You simply do not know what someone's health status is by looking at their size.

Aubrey Gordon, an author and podcaster, has spent years educating the public about the "widely documented substandard health care received by fat people, which can lead to postponement of care, misdiagnosis of crucial health conditions, and denial of care altogether."[1] Social prejudice against fat people, especially among medical professionals, has prevented countless patients from getting adequate medical care. In other words, the idea that being thin is healthy and being fat is unhealthy is not only overly simplistic; it puts real people at real risk of harm.

In *"You Just Need to Lose Weight" and 19 Other Myths About Fat People*, Gordon writes, "Whether being fat is a choice for an individual or not, they do not deserve discrimination, harassment, or unkind treatment because of the size of their bodies. None of us should have to change our appearance in order to 'earn' basic respect and dignity."[2]

Undoing our assumptions about what is "better" in terms of our bodies is a huge and extremely difficult process. It is personal, and it is likely lifelong, but it is also something we must engage in for our own and others' bodies, cultures, and communities to thrive.

Labeling bodies as good or bad perpetuates prejudice and unfair treatment in the aggregate, and self-abandonment at the personal level. We are much more likely to label our own bodies as bad than good. Self-abandonment is the key feature in our definition of addiction, and it is something trauma survivors know well.

Try this idea on: Your body is doing its absolute best to keep you alive and adjust to whatever is happening. There is no such thing as a correct or incorrect body. More on these ideas in the chapters to come.

Lie #3: Pleasure is not that important.

There are so many forms of pleasure that have been labeled as immoral, wrong, and sinful; perhaps "unimportant" seems like progress. Many women and gender-expansive people, especially those raised in socially conservative religions, already feel shame and guilt about their sexual feelings. Some, like Tamara, have had to leave the religion of their upbringing to feel free to pursue any pleasure with their chosen partners.

What Tamara has experienced, over the course of years after a traumatic car accident, is a slow deprioritizing of her own pleasure. Tamara doesn't feel that pleasure is available to her because she has chronic pain, is grieving her marriage, and struggles to care for her mother. Now, she is facing her own behavior and recognizing that her use of opioid pain medication is out of control. Among these concerns, pleasure seems unimportant. It seems silly or childish to her to try to find moments of joy or play in her life, period. Sexual pleasure seems a universe away.

Each person's definition of pleasure will be different, and it will change as they do. Sexual pleasure is only one of the infinite ways humans can experience enjoyment and awareness of the present moment. We have known many people who, for many reasons, no longer seek pleasure through sex. Some are asexual and do not experience sexual desire or arousal in a way that motivates them to seek sex. Some have used sexual relationships or sexual media in a way that became a problem in their lives, and they needed to stop. Some have had medical conditions that make sexual contact uncomfortable or infeasible.

Sexuality doesn't need to be the only or even the main source of pleasure in your life. But it is important to remember that pleasure is possible and that enjoying being alive is one good reason to live!

For people who struggle with addiction and compulsive behaviors, pleasure may feel like the origin of all our problems—didn't we enjoy drinking at first? Isn't pleasure-seeking the problem? If pleasure led us down the wrong path to begin with, de-emphasizing it can seem like the natural correction. Maybe we even believe we don't deserve to feel good ever again. Pleasure has to become less important to us if we are going to recover, right?

Crucially, no, pleasure itself is not the problem. We develop addictions and compulsive behavior as we seek to escape our pain and discomfort. However, relief from pain and discomfort is not the same thing as pleasure. Recovery is a process by which we begin to feel and understand the difference. When we seek to enjoy being alive in our body, and we want others around us to do the same, we can tap into pleasure rather than escape into temporary relief from suffering. Pleasure is important because it is an honest expression of ourselves. Sexual recovery is where all of these pieces come together.

Lie #4: Gender is irrelevant.

Many women find it difficult to recognize and accept sexism as a continuing, often thinly disguised fact of our lives. Others are deeply aware of it and wish they could forget about it. Transgender, nonbinary, and gender-diverse people all have specific viewpoints on how gender functions in our society and, ultimately, how much gender affects our lives.

In an interview with the BBC, Vivienne Ming, a trans woman and tech entrepreneur described a major difference she experienced after her transition. "Just overnight, people stopped asking me math questions," she says. The assumption, she explains, was that "maybe I was good at leading a project, but I surely couldn't understand the technical details behind it."[3]

Curious about how this social experience might translate into a material difference between men and women in the tech field, Ming conducted an experiment to calculate how much extra work women would need to do to get the same promotions as men. Ming's team found that women needed to go to better schools for longer and hold lower-status jobs for longer in order to achieve the same promotions as men in American tech companies. The cost to women? Approximately $250,000 over the course of a career. Ming calls it "the tax on being different."

Gender bias is everywhere, so it should be unsurprising that it ultimately affects every aspect of our lives. Realizing this can be disturbing, but it can also begin to connect you with your inner feelings about who you are and what sort of world you want to live in.

All cultures have some way of explaining sex and gender. The binary gender system we live in today is a construct built on what people observe about their bodies and behaviors, just like every other gender system has been. Prior to European colonization, there were many societies who interpreted sex and gender differently than our system does today. For example, in pre-contact Hawaii, Indigenous peoples honored a third gender, known as the māhū, translated today as "in the middle." The māhū were healers and culture workers, and there are Native Hawaiians today who carry on this tradition. Connection to the land, cultural tradition, language preservation, and family support to younger generations are all part of what the māhū provide in their communities.

Nova had an awakening about the importance of gender while in a group with other women in the adult industries. Growing up in a spiritual community, Nova had been taught that all people are equally beautiful and equally divine. She was taught that there were no real differences among people and that placing importance on things like race and gender was what caused wars, conflict, and pain.

Although many of her beliefs changed once she and her father had to leave the community, Nova was grateful to have been taught to value all human lives equally. It bothered her how much people seemed to care about her being a woman and also how much they cared about her skin color and her Mexican heritage. During a meeting with her group, Nova said maybe she would start using they/them pronouns for everyone, just because it leveled the playing field. A transgender woman in the group spoke up. "I use she/her," she said. "And I fought hard for my she/her, and I want you to use it."

Immediately, Nova understood that she had inadvertently made her friend uncomfortable. She had erased her friend's experience in trying to de-emphasize gender for herself. She did not mean to erase the real differences among her group members. Because she had internalized the sexism she experienced, Nova wanted to stop thinking about gender altogether, but that created a space where differences weren't celebrated either. Nova apologized and thought about that interaction often. Whenever she felt sick of "being a woman," she remembered that it was actually sexism she was sick of, not the fact of being herself.

If we hear powerful but unfair messages about gender repeated for ten, twenty, thirty, forty years, they become part of our consciousness. Their effect on our lives is enormous but often unexamined. Younger people today are still being profoundly affected by this aspect of the socialization process. It affects what we study, how we behave, what we wear, how we talk, whom we love. And it has a profound impact on the nature of our sexuality.

We must face the difficult reality that sexuality is impacted by gender violence. The statistics are chilling: Estimates range from one in nine to one in three American girls have been sexually abused before the age of eighteen; around 40 percent of adult women have been sexually harassed on the job; and one in five women will experience rape. These statistics are even higher if the woman has an alcohol or substance use disorder. Rates of violence and sexual assault are also higher for queer, transgender, and nonbinary people.

As we begin to reconnect with who we really are, who we want to be, and how we want to be in community with others, we must keep our eye on creating safety for ourselves and others, honoring each person's experience of their body, gender, and sexuality. Cultivating pleasure and honoring our authentic selves can be an act of liberation.

Lie #5: There is an ideal way to be sexual, and you are failing at it. In our sexual lives, as in every other part of our lives, when we deny the reality of our feelings, we relinquish our power of discretion and our power of choice. To recover our power, we must give voice to our fear, grief, joy, desire, and curiosity.

The first step is to concentrate on finding your voice. Most of us have had little practice talking about sexual issues. It can seem embarrassing and intrusive, but sharing ideas and experiences about sexuality with trusted people who are ready to listen and communicate can be a healing experience. You may learn things about yourself you never suspected, and you will begin to appreciate the experiences of others, both similar and dissimilar to your own.

If you do not feel comfortable connecting with a group at first, you can start by talking with a close friend. If that also feels too uncomfortable, you may want to begin by reading or watching educational material on sexuality. If you have the means to seek out sex therapy, you can consult listings for therapists with expertise in your area, like the database at *Psychology Today*.

Begin wherever you can; begin where you are. Begin right here in this book, and imagine that you are not failing at sexuality; you are taking action toward a sexual life that reflects your personality, values, and joys. Changes like this always seem to move slower than we wish they would, so be patient and gentle with yourself. There will always be challenges.

When co-author Vanessa told their parents that they were queer, and in love with a woman and a man at the same time, their parents' first response was sadness. "You are going to have a very hard life," they said. This reinforced an underlying belief that it is better to be heterosexual and monogamous, maybe not because it is wrong to be queer and nonmonogamous, but because it is "harder." But why is being queer so hard? Is it not because of social prejudice and structural barriers?

Years later, Vanessa processed this moment with a therapist who encouraged Vanessa to imagine a response that contained more joy about who they are. What could Vanessa's parents have said that might indicate their support, rather than their fear of the hardships Vanessa might encounter?

Vanessa wrote down some ideas. "We are so lucky to have you in our family!" "Thank you for trusting us with this truth; we will put in some time and self-educate so we can support you the best way possible!" "You are not alone; we will be right beside you as you grow." Imagining this kind of support allowed Vanessa to release some of the shame and sadness they felt. When connecting with their partners, Vanessa felt freer to express their happiness.

If your sexual life is unsatisfactory to you right now, and you are concerned that you are doing something wrong, take heart. Whether you are having less sexual connection than you'd prefer, like Michelle and Tamara, or feel the need to back off and reevaluate your sexual preferences and sources of pleasure, like Ash and Nova, you are doing it right. You can change direction at any time, even if you have a long-term partner. Your sexuality is for you to experiment with, learn about, be friends with, and find pleasure in, at your own pace. You are in charge of your awakening.

The Hope of Truth

Women in recovery almost unanimously express dissatisfaction with their sexual lives, but there are precious few tools available to help sort out our discomfort. Sometimes we hide our unhappiness and disappointment, avoiding the topic altogether. Sometimes we are stoic about the dreariness of our sex lives. Sometimes we are angry and resentful because we aren't having the kind of sexual experiences that we want. Sometimes we feel so grateful to be sober that we pretend we can live without other pleasures—like a satisfying sex life. Rarely do we have the opportunity in treatment programs, in Twelve Step meetings, or in therapy to talk about our sexual dissatisfactions unless we seek out programs that are specifically designed for this purpose.

The first step in a sexual recovery process is to be honest about your sexual feelings, whether they are clear or cloudy, familiar or new. Being honest takes courage and the willingness to find out what it is that you want and feel, and to discover a way to express it.

The tools provided here are designed to allow you to discover your sexual feelings, and to bring your actions into congruence with those feelings. Not all the exercises emphasize sexual touch, because connecting with sexuality might also ask us to connect with our body more generally. For example, we may need to do some healing around our body image or develop more comfort with nonsexual touch first.

If you find it difficult to express or receive nonsexual touch and affection, friendship and companionship can be places where profound healing takes place. We may be developing a language of affection with a partner at the same time that we develop a language of sexual pleasure on our own. There is no wrong way to proceed, as long as you are moving intentionally, gently, and with honesty.

Becoming who you want to be sexually is about becoming whole; it is about becoming a person with choice, empowered to risk and change. It is about integrating your feelings and actions into a seamless web of self, bridging the gap between your inner feelings and your outer actions. It is about rekindling your inner light and letting it shine. It is about finding wholeness and consciously welcoming into being the person you already are.

○ ○ ○

CHAPTER 3

The Flow of Desire and Pleasure

Desire is not simply a desire of each self for its self-pleasure. But what is it for?

Possibly, if it is for anything, desire is for the experience of the journey toward and joining in something that thereby becomes greater than the separate selves. Desire in the larger sense affirms our connection and being "a part of" rather than "apart from." It leads to expansion rather than satisfaction; the former suggests growth, life, and openness; the latter suggests stasis.

———

Judith V. Jordan, "Clarity in Connection: Empathic Knowing, Desire, and Sexuality"

S exual desire describes the powerful, potent mix of sexual urges, stirrings, and interests that we feel. We may express them toward a potential or current lover. Even though we hear desire discussed freely and can recognize it in others, the experience of desire can be confusing: sometimes elusive, sometimes overwhelming. This is especially true for people as they recover from the emotional, physical, and psychological consequences of addiction and trauma. Knowing when you feel desire and being relatively comfortable expressing it are vital steps on your journey toward sexual empowerment, but that's only the beginning.

Importantly, an overemphasis on feeling sexual desire can backfire. This is because sexual desire waxes and wanes based on many factors, some under our control, many not. Your sexuality may involve a lot of *spontaneous desire:* You may see a sexy person in the grocery store and instantly fantasize about their naked body. You may consistently want sex with your current or potential partners. Or you may require more context, more attention, and more pleasure before your desire emerges—this is called *responsive desire*. Most people tend toward one type or the other, spontaneous or responsive, and it is normal to experience them both. It is also normal to feel neither! It doesn't mean you are unable to feel pleasure.

The only form of desire our culture seems to care about is spontaneous desire, and it is presumed to be part of a "normal" sexual life. The truth is, no matter how much or how little spontaneous desire you feel, your unique sexuality can respond to pleasure. This chapter will help you understand your patterns from the past, identify challenges you may face in experiencing desire and pleasure, and empower you to seek the pleasure that works for you.

What Is Desire?

Poets, painters, dancers, doctors, therapists . . . it seems everyone has weighed in on this question. People have too much or too little, are consumed by it, or long to feel it again. We will join an increasing number of voices in the sexuality field when we say that desire is more complex than we've been led to believe. Every human experiences it differently, and some find they don't experience it at all. And this variety is healthy, normal, acceptable, and inevitable.

There is no wrong way to feel desire—you may feel it at inopportune times, for inappropriate people, quietly or loudly, quickly or slowly, like a lightning strike or a slow creep of lava. Perhaps you are more likely to feel desire after touching or kissing someone, or after a particularly insightful and stimulating conversation. Maybe you desire only one person at a time, or maybe you feel a desire to jump into bed with anyone who has that one haircut. Your desire can take many shapes. The idea that there is one right way to experience desire (spontaneously, at the sight of a partner!) is not only unhelpful; it creates a lot of shame and stress.

While spontaneous desire can be extremely compelling, you may notice we are not using the word *need* or *drive* to describe it. The feeling of sexual desire is not the same thing as the hard-wired need for companionship with other humans, something researchers have demonstrated over and over again. Humans need to be around other humans to be well. At the same time, no single human needs sex with any other human, the way humans need air, food, water, warmth, sleep, and other humans around to survive.

For those of us who have been pressured into sex we didn't want because of someone else's "need": They and their untruth abused us. For those of us who pressured others into sex because of how powerfully we felt desire: We were behaving abusively. Many of us have experienced both roles. Our recovery requires us to acknowledge that sexual desire does not give anyone a right to pressure someone. Sexual desire is a set of feelings and sensations, an internal experience. Sexual pressure is a behavior, an external experience.

Developing a comprehensive model of human sexual desire has been a complex problem for researchers. For decades, desire has been pathologized as either too low or too high, diagnosable as a problem but rarely met with real solutions. This is because the state of perfect spontaneous desire is an illusion, a socially constructed chimera.

There are ways to open the door for more desire if that is what you want, and we will discuss them. But keep in mind: Desire is only one piece of the puzzle when it comes to sexuality, and it changes throughout your life, over a month, sometimes within a day.

What if there was nothing wrong with how you feel or don't feel desire? What if the fantasies you entertain inside your mind and body are totally allowed there? What if having no fantasies at all was also perfectly acceptable? What if your capacity to experience pleasure was not predicted by how much or how little spontaneous desire you feel? Take a moment with these questions, and imagine how you might feel.

Some sexuality therapy books define *sexual desire* as the specific sensations that push us to seek out or become receptive to sexual experiences. Unfortunately, that description of desire may not be helpful to us. We may seek out or become receptive to sexual experiences for many reasons other than desire.

Nova, for example, learned to use her sexual attractiveness to make a living as a dancer in a strip club. When she had sex with men outside the club during her active addiction, it wasn't important whether she actually desired the man or the sexual experience. She became an expert at pleasing men; she was alert and responsive to their sexual needs and desires, but she did not know what pleased her or whether she was feeling sexual desire. Her body's signals were often unclear, especially when she was using alcohol, cocaine, and methamphetamine, but she still wasn't sure how much desire she was feeling even after she got sober.

Nova did maintain some boundaries, even at the apex of her addiction. She remembers saying no to a few men who physically repulsed her. "But most of them were fine with me," she muses, "it's just, my standards are changing now that I'm sober."

Nova remembers feeling curious about sex as a child, and she misses the feeling of playful experimentation that characterized her life in the large community where she grew up. Because she has so much sexual experience, she doesn't think of herself as needing to "discover" her body or sexuality; instead, she says she wants to reconnect with her own innate sense of desire. She wants to have a clearer separation between the clients she entertains as a dancer and the people she has sexual relationships with for herself.

In her support group, a sex worker friend tells Nova she understands where Nova is coming from. "Sometimes my whole sex life is just client sex," she says. "I need to make money, but eventually you need a break to recenter and listen to your own body for a while." Curious about this idea, Nova decided to try a three-month experiment: no sex with anyone except herself.

Nova continued to work at the club, where she has made a living for six years and has a dedicated group of regular customers. She announced on her social media that she was going to do a celibacy experiment and received mixed responses. Some supported her, as they had since the beginning of her recovery. Others told her celibacy is "unnatural" and that she is going against a biological drive. For Nova, deciding to stop having sex with other people for a while felt like turning down a noisy stereo, and she was curious about what she might discover about herself.

Soon, Nova started connecting more consciously with her own pleasure and arousal, and with the help of her support group, she was able to speak authentically about her experiments. She methodically attempted to find new pleasures for every one of her five senses. She bought a new, soft blanket that she loves to touch. She lit candles in her room instead of turning on the overhead light to delight her vision. When she started seeking pleasure for her sense of taste, however, she hit a snag.

Nova discovered that her relationship with food had been disordered ever since she got sober. While she was getting high, she easily maintained extreme thinness because she rarely felt hungry. Once she decided she needed to maintain sobriety, she began restricting her food, afraid of gaining weight. "I have to stay in form," she would tell herself, "or I'll lose my job."

Like many women who quit using amphetamines, Nova gained weight in sobriety, weight that was actually a sign of health. She kept her body under strict control to minimize the changes, pinching herself unconsciously and disapproving of her body in the mirror, while feeling increasingly ashamed of her own negativity. She felt she was supposed to be confident, but she wasn't anymore. Everything she ate made her feel guilty, and she stopped eating the foods that she used to find most delicious, because they were "bad."

As she began experimenting with finding new pleasures for her five senses, the lack of enjoyment she felt eating food, and the way she was restricting herself, was clearer. Nova knew that the pressure on her to maintain her body shape and weight was going to be intense, as long as she was trying to make money as a dancer. Within that pressure, she wanted to find a way to eat regular, healthy meals.

She felt scared and stuck, just like she had at the beginning of getting sober. Still, she knew she had reached a new place in her recovery. "I want to want good food," she wrote in her journal. "I want to enjoy tastes and textures and feel like food can be a pleasure, not a threat. I want to be okay with what happens to my body when I eat."

Nova applied her recovery principles to this exploration and began educating herself on anorexia and attending an online support group for people recovering from eating disorders. What surprised Nova the most during these months was how strongly she started craving methamphetamine again. A year ago, she had been able to reduce her use and then quit altogether without medical intervention, although her first few weeks sober had been difficult. She had been exhausted, anxious, and depressed, but she had friends helping her along the way who had experience, and she was able to make it through.

Now, a year later, she was struggling in a new way as she addressed the symptoms of her disordered eating. She had been able to push through the difficulty of sobriety with her tenacity and self-awareness. This new phase would require additional skills: gentleness, self-compassion, and curiosity. Nova's desire to experience pleasure through her senses guided her to another level of recovery.

You do not need to experience spontaneous sexual desire to be able to experience pleasure. Your desire can take the form of seeking new ways to connect with your own body and feel the sensations that delight you. The more you notice what pleases you, the more you can cultivate those pleasures. Let your desire for connection and knowledge of self be your guide.

EXERCISE

Engaging the Senses

The following exercise is designed to aid you in reconnecting to the power of your body's senses.

Every day for the next five days, do your best to notice the information your senses bring to you.

- **Day One:** Focus on your sight. What do you see? Notice if it pleases you, seems beautiful, or piques your curiosity.

- **Day Two:** Focus on your hearing. What sounds do you notice in your daily life? Which ones are pleasing, and which ones are grating to you? Can you cultivate more pleasant sounds, like playing music or listening to birds in the morning?

- **Day Three:** Focus on your senses of smell and taste. They are deeply linked, and noticing this link is part of the practice. What scents and smells do you notice? Are they pleasant for you? Do any of them make your mouth

- water? How does your food smell, and how does it taste? Take some time to notice.

- **Day Four:** Focus on your sense of touch. Notice the textures you are in contact with. Where do you feel softness, ridges, sharp edges, hard surfaces? Which textures are you most interested in?

- **Day Five:** Focus on *interoception*, or sensing inside your body. Throughout the day, check in with your body on the inside. How is your throat, stomach, lower gut? Where do you feel muscle tension, and where do you feel relaxation?

Tuning in to our senses in this way can help us stay in the present moment. It can help us build up our capacity to enjoy what our bodies perceive and give us information about what we like and don't like in our environment. Tuning in to the inside of your body is a great way to reconnect with your inner sensations, which can open doors to your erotic experience. Some even find these exercises spark more spontaneous sexual desire!

Understanding Sexual Arousal

Arousal, pleasure, and desire have an intricate relationship, but they are not the same.

In her groundbreaking book *Come As You Are: The Surprising New Science That Will Transform Your Sex Life*,[1] Dr. Emily Nagoski dove into the science of desire, arousal, pleasure, and orgasm. She introduced much of the world to the *dual control model*, which was originally developed at the Kinsey Institute in the 1990s by Erick Janssen and John Bancroft. What is important about this model is that it goes beyond the basics of what happens to our bodies—vaginal lubrication, erection of the clitoris, erection of the penis, and so on—to give us a fuller picture of arousal. For those who are interested in the science of sexuality, Nagoski's work is a great place to begin.

Very briefly, the dual control model describes sexual arousal as a system that has both an accelerator and a brake, like a car. They are separate functions, the brake and the accelerator, and every person is going to have different levels of sensitivity in each. A person with a sensitive accelerator may feel turned on easily, but if they also have a sensitive brake, they can be turned off just as quickly. Sometimes, both seem to happen simultaneously.

According to Nagoski, it is most common for women to be somewhere in the middle level of sensitivity in both their accelerator and their brake. Also, she notes that all of this research has been done on women who were born with female anatomy, and we do not currently have strong research on the ways transgender women may be the same or different. However, it shouldn't be surprising that addiction, compulsive behaviors, and traumatic experiences can powerfully affect anyone's accelerating and braking systems. (So can many mood-stabilizing medications, giving birth, menopause, gender transition, and so much more.)

What hits your brake on any given day will be predicted by context—how you are feeling that day, how things feel between you and your partner, how stressed you are about your kids, or work, or paying a bill, or avoiding alcohol. Same goes for the accelerator. For some people, the accelerator is activated the instant they see their lover walk through the door. For others, the accelerator may respond to receiving a thoughtful card, physical touch, an hour of quiet, a delicious meal, the resolution of a conflict, a sexy scene in a movie—the list goes on. If something takes pressure off your brake, like having all the chores done, it can make room for your accelerator to really motivate sexual arousal.

Understanding that we all have both an accelerator and a brake can help us let go of the expectation of continuous spontaneous desire, and it can help us be gentler with ourselves if our body isn't responding the way we want it to. Women and gender-diverse people who have experienced sexual trauma may have the brake on more than others, because sexual feelings ignite feelings of fear or lack of safety. It is also possible that survivors of sexual trauma may have a very active accelerator, which can contribute to taking more sexual risks, even feeling out of control with sexual behavior.

What is at work in your own body as you recover? What hits your accelerator now? What hits your brake? What might hit them at the same time? Some people find that feeling upset hits their accelerator, and for others it hits the brake.

For those of us in recovery, heightened states of feeling, such as the excitement at meeting a new, sexy person or the pressure to excel at a new job, can activate both the accelerator and the brake at the same time, and we need some space and self-compassion to sort out our confusion. Like Daniel Tiger from *Daniel Tiger's Neighborhood* says, "Sometimes you feel two feelings at the same time, and that's okay."

Honesty without judgment is crucial when investigating yourself here. Many of us have stayed in relationships that were full of conflict because the conflict seemed like it hit our accelerator, and the makeup sex was a torrent of passion. The idealization of dramatic reconciliation is all around us. We may only get aroused when there is some drama afoot. If this is you, be assured that there are ways you can create some adrenaline in your sex life safely, in time.

Another feature of arousal we must be aware of as we continue talking about sexuality is known as *arousal nonconcordance*. Sexuality researchers have spent decades investigating the way bodies become aroused, often drawing the conclusion that a person's genitals tell a different story than their words do. Why does this happen?

Dr. Emily Nagoski reassures us that arousal nonconcordance happens when our body's response to something does not match our feelings, and it is *totally normal*. Sexual imagery or stimuli may lead to a genital response, but only the person having the experience can tell you if they feel turned on or not. Your genital response is not the "truth" of arousal; your subjective experience is.

Physiological sexual arousal may include increased blood flow to the skin and genitals, lubrication of the vagina, increased respiration and heart rate, and a host of other changes. However, if a person is simultaneously experiencing a sense that they do not want to have a sexual experience right now, that emotional experience should take priority. It works the other direction too. Perhaps someone wants to be sexual with herself or a partner, but because her vagina isn't "wet enough," she is discouraged and thinks maybe she was wrong about her desire. She wasn't wrong; she was just experiencing some arousal nonconcordance.

Arousal nonconcordance is an especially important concept for survivors of sexual trauma. Many women and gender-diverse people feel shame about how their body responded while they were being assaulted. A genital response during an assault does not mean the survivor enjoyed the experience. It means their body noticed something sex-related was happening and responded to that mechanically—not out of desire or pleasure. The emotional experience of sexual violation is not undermined by a nonconcordant physical response. Physical arousal can be deeply connected to pleasure and desire, but it can also be elusive—happening without pleasure, or not happening when we are sure we are feeling desire.

If your own body seems mystifying, unpredictable, or non-concordant in response to the world around you, you are in good company. The more time you spend listening to your own feelings and caring for your body, the easier it will be for you to know what actually feels good to you and what you want. Arousal nonconcordance may still happen, but it will be less distressing because you know it is a normal experience.

Physical and Emotional Challenges

Virtually all people are capable of feeling pleasure. Sexual pleasure may be more difficult for people in recovery for a host of reasons. Some include the physical challenges of recovery, such as returning to health after withdrawal, and some may be seen as more emotional challenges, such as processing loss and grief. Physical and emotional challenges are deeply interconnected. Emotions are a physical experience, and physical experiences affect our emotions.

Early recovery can be a time of stress and crisis. Recovery brings change, and even positive change is stressful. Stress affects our ability to feel pleasure. It can be helpful to remember that stress is a bodily experience, and that you can support your own body's ability to metabolize stress. This begins with attending to basic needs: moving your body regularly, eating nourishing food, and getting plenty of rest. As your recovery progresses, you should find that the number of crises in your life reduces. At the same time, you will develop more skills and tools for handling stress. This will open up more capacity for pleasure and connection.

What follows is a list of common challenges many women, nonbinary people, and gender-expansive people experience when they begin the work of recovering sexually. These challenges will intertwine and intersect differently for each person, and they can be affected by any of the intersecting identities we've mentioned: age, race, size, disability, and so on. While each of these challenges requires care and attention, none of them mean you are incapable of experiencing sexual pleasure.

Ebb and Flow of Desire

No one has the same level of sexual interest all the time. If you have a trusting relationship, and there is no unresolved conflict, then you may simply be in a period of low sexual interest, without there being a problem to solve. Throughout our lives we feel an ebb and flow of our desire, just as we do with other forms of physical or intellectual energy. At some points in our lives we may feel more sexual and have more interest in being sexual; at others, less. This constant ebb and flow is natural and normal.

Your level of sexual interest may be related to your hormonal cycle; it may be greatly affected by pregnancy, nursing, and menopause. Sometimes it is related to a fear of unwanted pregnancy. Many women report that menopause was a sexually freeing experience for them, and that desire flowered after fifty. Some women report that their desire increased with age, as they felt more secure in their bodies and less self-conscious. Other women say that their sexual response mellowed and became less insistent with age. Some women report desire as less genitally focused and more diffuse with age, and others say the opposite. There is no one right way to experience the changes that our lives will bring.

Health Concerns in Early Alcohol/Substance Use Recovery

Many women experience a decrease in sexual desire during the first two years of sobriety. Early recovery can be an intense time, requiring you to mobilize all your resources. You may simply not have the energy available for sexual interests. We have heard many clients echo the sentiments of this recovering woman with alcohol use disorder: "I was exhausted when I quit drinking.

All I wanted to do was sleep. I had zero interest in sex. I felt like I was recovering from a long illness."

Women in early recovery have to deal with the physical effects of their alcohol or substance use, eating disorders, and other forms of self-neglect. The physical effects can be serious, and some may require ongoing support.

Sexual feelings of desire and pleasure are most available when we are feeling safe, comfortable in our bodies, and open to connection. During early recovery, we may be involved in the process of regaining our health and energy. We have to establish new patterns around meeting our own basic needs. Eating regular meals, sleeping without first getting drunk or high, and replacing compulsive behaviors with more self-supportive activity is a giant set of tasks.

Some women have exhausted their adrenal glands and experience a deep sense of fatigue. Others will be healing from ulcers, respiratory ailments, or the effect of alcohol on the liver. Many of our addictive substances and behaviors changed the baseline chemistry in our brains, and we simply may not be able to find our sexual arousal accelerator for a time.

Depending on what behaviors or substances we are recovering from, we may need to be patient and consistent in rebuilding as much health as we can before we think about sex.

Perhaps, like Nova, you need more time than you thought to attend to your basic needs. Or maybe, like Tamara, you need to accept that your body and your life have already changed, and you need to care for yourself in this new moment rather than try to "get back to normal." Whatever was normal in the past is no longer available, and it is time to build a new normal. With time and tenacity, that new normal can feel much better than anything we had before, even with the changes we may have gone through.

Gynecological Issues

People with vulvas benefit greatly from regular gynecological care. Getting that care is challenging enough for cisgender women, nearly half of whom avoid their yearly pelvic exam. It is more difficult still for trans women who have had genital reconstructive surgery, nonbinary people assigned female at birth, trans men who have not had genital reconstructive surgery, intersex people, and other gender-expansive people to find doctors with whom they can be comfortable and trusting. But take heart, as there are more trauma-informed and gender-inclusive doctors being minted every day, who are making regular gynecological care easier to adhere to.

Women with alcohol use disorder (AUD) experience more gynecological difficulties during both active drinking and recovery than women without AUD. Be mindful of an increased risk of bacterial vaginosis (BV), which has been associated with heavy drinking.[2] While research is ongoing, we still do not know all the mechanisms by which alcohol and other drugs affect our reproductive systems.

Anecdotally, we know that the easier it is to access sexual and reproductive health care, the more patients will seek it, even if they are engaged in higher-risk behaviors with substances. If a kind and competent doctor is close by, and making an appointment is simple, and the treatments are affordable, it makes sense that more people would find their way into a doctor's office.

If in-person care is not easily accessible, or if you'd prefer to begin by asking your questions online, many websites and apps are available to help. Always check to make sure that your sources of information have appropriate credentials. Many women's health practitioners are creating newsletters, free videos, and accessible websites to help answer common questions.

Untreated issues, like endometriosis, polycystic ovarian syndrome (PCOS), and fibroids, can contribute to intense pelvic pain, heavy periods, digestive disturbance, and a host of other symptoms that can leave you feeling less than sexy. In early recovery, it's important to get a thorough pelvic exam, complete with tests for common sexually transmitted infections (STIs, also known as STDs). Ask for a referral in your community, as the women around you are the best resource for referrals to a doctor in your area who has experience with trauma, substance use disorders, eating disorders, and so on.

Pain with sex is a common experience, and having an exam to rule out infections or other conditions will help you make a plan for reducing discomfort and increasing pleasure. Many people find that using more lubrication does the trick, but of course that is not always the only answer. If you are experiencing pain with penetration, are having some trouble holding in your pee when you sneeze or laugh, have a history of bladder prolapse, or have another issue related to your pelvic floor, there is more support available now than for generations past.

Once major medical issues have been ruled out, a pelvic floor physical therapist can do an exam specifically to assess your body and make recommendations for you. This may include the use of dilators for vaginismus, a condition in which the vagina involuntarily contracts, which is a common diagnosis for survivors of sexual trauma. Another option is a pelvic trigger point wand, which can help to release scar tissue, a common issue for those who have given birth.

Linda, who had been in recovery since her early thirties, was diagnosed with cervical and vaginal cancer at sixty years old. She went through several rounds of treatment, and a large tumor was removed from her vagina. In order to do this, her surgeon had to remove most of her vagina as well. Linda healed well, but vaginal penetration was no longer an option. Because she had already experienced menopause, she felt as if her doctors had assumed she was no longer sexually active with her husband, or that somehow it wouldn't be a big issue for her.

She was angry, sad, and frustrated that her doctors had not prepared her for this outcome. Although she was cancer-free, Linda became depressed, and this led to a return to alcohol use, the first she'd had for decades.

But Linda was determined to live *and* to experience pleasure. She found a support group for cancer survivors and returned to sobriety. Linda and her husband, who had been sexually active together up until her cancer symptoms became too painful, entered couple's counseling with a sex therapist to process what was happening. They grieved the loss of a sexual activity that had brought them both years of pleasure and connection. They worried about whether they would be able to feel the same level of intimacy without penetrative sex.

The sex therapist worked with them to establish new ways of connecting sexually, with a focus on the pleasures that were still available to them, as well as some new ones they had never thought to try. The therapist also referred Linda to a pelvic floor physical therapist, who helped her heal from her surgery, strengthen her muscles, and release tension from the physical trauma and scarring. While vaginal penetration was still not an option for her, Linda was eventually able to find her way to a new, different, but still-vibrant sexual life with her husband. This would not have happened if she hadn't asked for support, advocated for her sexuality, and found the right team.

Unresolved Conflict

For many recovering couples, unexpressed anger and unresolved conflict are major blocks to the flow of desire and pleasure.

In our work with clients, we have heard many people express variations of the following statements:

- "My partner doesn't listen to me, hear me, or see me anymore. Why would I want sex with them?"
- "My boyfriend stares at his phone all night, not saying a word. Then I'm supposed to suddenly feel sexual just because we're in bed together? That's not how it works."
- "I thought my recovery might inspire her, but she's still actively drinking/using and it turns me off."
- "I can't feel sexy on the spur of the moment. I need to feel intimate before I feel desire. No one I meet wants to wait until the third or fourth date like I do."
- "He touches me for three minutes in the way that's fun for him and expects me to be aroused. He doesn't understand that sex isn't something he does to me; it's something that we could be doing together."
- "I don't feel full of desire after we've been bickering and fighting all day, but she does."
- "Bad sex isn't worth wanting."

All of these statements imply some conflict between partners. If you are having difficulty experiencing sexual connection with a current partner, then it is important to look first at the relationship. If you do not feel close and trusting, or if you have trouble communicating, then your brake may be on far more than your accelerator can compensate for. This was certainly the case for Michelle and Chris, who struggled to connect because of the unresolved conflict they were in about Michelle's drinking, substance use, and overspending.

Establishing communication about sex early in a dating relationship can reduce confusion and anxiety, but it does require a special set of skills: emotional self-regulation, the ability to communicate with compassion and curiosity, and sexual self-awareness. We will spend more time on this in chapters 7 and 11.

Sexual Abuse

In our experience working with clients, the number one impediment to sexual desire and pleasure is a history of sexual or physical abuse. Women who have been raped, sexually abused in childhood, beaten, or violated another way may then connect sex or touching with pain and fear, guilt and shame. This is a natural reaction. It is also common for survivors to go to the other extreme and become sexually active far beyond what is pleasurable or desirable for them.

Ash's response to the childhood sexual abuse they experienced from their stepfather was to become hypersexual. As a young adult entering a recovery program for the first time, Ash felt intense internal conflict about their sexual behavior, so they didn't reveal much to their first sponsor in AA. Outside of their sober community, Ash was part of a queer, sex-positive group of friends, and Ash didn't want to be perceived as slut-shaming anyone, including themself.

"I saw it all in very simplistic terms," Ash remembers. "Lots of sex was supposed to be good, and I'd had lots of sex, but I didn't feel good about it, so something had to be wrong with me." Ash returned to using heroin and other substances more than once because the shame and pain they experienced was so persistent.

It wasn't having lots of sex that was the problem—people can have sex with multiple partners in a joyful way if they are choosing to do so. The issue was how Ash approached sex, which was more compulsively, as a means to an end, and the end was never fully achieved. They were never satisfied, never loved enough, never safe enough, and never cared for enough, even though sex would often help them meet a need or two for a short time.

If you are a survivor of sexual violence or physical abuse, it is important to get counseling with a professional who is trained to work with trauma. Many of us feel a strong need to be heard, seen, and validated in our experience. Identifying and recalling details of violence and abuse can cause us to reexperience the old feelings of pain and shame, numbness, lack of connection, or rage. There are strategies to help you cope with these effects, should you choose to tell your stories. Containment in a therapeutic environment is one of them.

At the same time, recent research has suggested that some trauma survivors fare better without recalling the details of their experience, as long as they are consistently engaged with body-based practices that help them feel safer with others, in the present moment. Somatic—also known as body-based—practices can take many forms, such as eye movement desensitization and reprocessing (EMDR), Somatic Experiencing (SE), and other somatic therapies. The first step is self-regulation: tuning into what is happening in our bodies, feeling the feelings that are arising, and allowing them to pass through. The second step is developing positive social connections that encourage us to feel seen, heard, and safe.

This is a change in therapeutic wisdom from most of the twentieth century, in which psychologists were trained to help women share memories of abuse. The standard of care for trauma was several forms of talk therapy, where the story of the abuse may be told multiple times. Again, for some, this may be a helpful practice, but we do have more options today.

According to Dr. Bruce Perry, a trauma and resilience researcher and author, "The most powerful buffer in times of stress and distress is our social connectedness."[3] Dr. Perry and other trauma specialists suggest that the therapeutic value of physical activity like dance, martial arts, yoga, and walking with a friend can be enormous, because patterned, rhythmic, repetitive movement helps us self-regulate, and sharing these practices with a trusted friend or in a group helps us form more positive social relationships.

If you have a history of sexual trauma or physical violence, we strongly urge you to spend some time deliberately addressing your history with a method, practitioner, or group that feels like the right fit for you. Your individual somatic practice and your therapeutic social connections do not need to happen at the same time, but keeping an eye out for ways to integrate them can be deeply beneficial.

Mental Health Challenges: Depression, Anxiety, Post-Traumatic Stress, and More

As the field of clinical psychology develops its understanding of trauma, many diagnoses, including depression, anxiety, and post-traumatic stress disorder, have made their way into more mainstream conversations. Influencers on social media are naming many behaviors "a trauma response." Terms like *triggers* and *flashbacks*, which do have specific meanings in the therapy context, are used publicly to refer to a host of uncomfortable experiences. This mainstreaming of psychological language is neither good nor bad; it is just a change that has occurred in the past ten years that can affect how we evaluate our own emotional lives.

It may be difficult to know for yourself if what you are experiencing now is related to traumatic experiences in your past, and how much your past has shaped your current relationships with other people, your own body, your substances, and your behaviors. When we feel distress, we ask *why?* And for many of us, a diagnosis and treatment program can help us make sense of what we are going through.

For some, however, diagnoses are not helpful, and the mental health care system where they are decided and treated is not a safe place to process emotional experience. As people with significant experience in these systems, we see how receiving a diagnosis can relieve suffering for one while causing more suffering to another.

What is most important is that you are staying true to your own values and beliefs about what emotional health looks like for you. If you are experiencing symptoms that are interfering with your daily life, seeking mental health care may be an important next step. Crucially, any mental health challenge will likely affect your sexuality in one way or another.

Depression often has a negative effect on sexual desire, one widely demonstrated in studies of all types of people. Losing interest in pleasurable activities is one of the most-often reported criteria for a diagnosis of depression. Depression is often related to feelings of powerlessness, helplessness, and unexpressed anger. We can feel this way when we see no options for ourselves and feel trapped in our life situations. It is not uncommon for people who have been sober for a few months to experience increased anxiety and depression. If the substance or behavior that was numbing our distress is withdrawn, eventually our distress will make itself known.

You may feel almost continually depressed, down, and sad, or you may feel "blue" for a few days or weeks at a time, with more or less normal periods in between. You may want to get a diagnostic evaluation, especially if you are experiencing suicidal thoughts, engaging in self-harm, or engaging in other behavior that causes danger or distress to the people around you. Individual and group therapy can often help us see possibilities for change that we weren't aware of.

It may feel like a cruel irony, then, to experience sexual side effects from a medication that helps with depression. The most common sexual side effects are lack of sexual interest and difficulty with orgasm, so if you decide to take medication for depression, do keep an eye on how it affects your sexual feelings. Sexual side effects can usually be managed, but you do have to tell your prescribing doctor about them. Sometimes they decrease over the first six months on a new medication. Sometimes they are treated with another medication, and sometimes they can be alleviated with a more patient approach to sexual activity, such as more time spent warming your body up to sexual touch.

Anxiety, post-traumatic stress disorder, acute stress disorder, and other diagnoses that have a direct relationship with trauma can all interfere with how we experience our bodies, our relationships, and our ability to sexually connect. Symptoms that arise during sexual experiences, like going numb or dissociating when a partner initiates sex, are common responses to sexual trauma. For those with sexual trauma, mental health symptoms are often a signal that sexual recovery is needed.

Mental health concerns require daily care and attention so we can rebuild our inner sense of safety. Sexual safety cannot be built from an emotional world where no safety is available. The goal is not to be rid of our capacity to feel deeply; the goal is to become both deeply feeling and deeply connected to others, supported by and supportive to those we love.

Loss and Grief

Loss and grief have an impact on every facet of our lives. It is common for women in early recovery to experience grief over the loss of their substance or behavior as their constant companion and comfort. Recovering people may feel they have lost years of their lives to addiction or compulsivity, and as they return to health they may need to face many accompanying losses: loss of memory, loss of adolescence, loss of career, loss of loved ones, loss of self-worth. Grief is a complex, enormous part of the human experience, and it deserves proper time, care, and support. Many people will avoid feeling grief as much as they can, afraid that if they open the door, they may never be able to stop crying.

In her book *It's OK That You're Not OK: Meeting Grief and Loss in a Culture That Doesn't Understand*, Megan Devine writes that "grief no more needs a solution than love needs a solution." Grief is powerful because it is part of how we process our love for other people and our attachments in our own lives. It can be a painful, exhausting physical experience.

During the process of grieving, many people experience very little sexual pleasure and an almost total loss of sexual interest. This is a common experience during any grieving process, whether for the loss of another person or for the loss of parts of yourself.

It is also normal, however, for people to go to the opposite extreme and feel an increase in spontaneous sexual desire while processing grief and loss. Neither response is good nor bad. They both require gentleness, self-awareness, and support.

As you work through your recovery, grief will continue to be your companion. We do not solve, banish, or fix it. We learn to accept and tend to it. We encourage you to make sure you have support as you allow its waves of intensity to wash over you. The only thing we can promise is that time will pass, and so if you practice being more present with your grief starting now, you will be able to build the emotional self-care skills you need as you move forward in your life.

Seeking Pleasure

As you become more stable and well in your recovery, you will probably experience a gradual increase in your sexual interest. If you do not, there are a number of steps you can take to create more safety for your pleasure to emerge.

Remember that sexual recovery is not a linear process. It can help to think of it more like an upward spiral (see Figure 1). You will likely return to many of the same issues, memories, and questions you had at the beginning of your recovery, but in more nuanced ways, with more skills to navigate them, and with a greater sense of who you are and where you are headed. As you put in the work and move up the spiral over time, you will transform, and more pleasure and connection will become available to you.

FIGURE 1

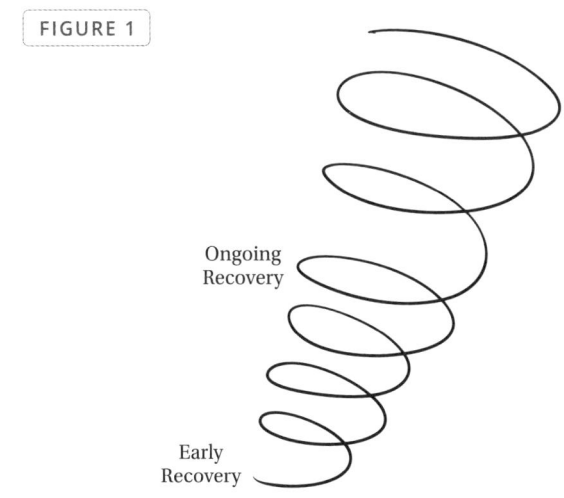

Ongoing
Recovery

Early
Recovery

If you are in a partnership, you may need to get more comfortable talking about sex: what it means to you, what you want from it, how it feels to you. This is a basic part of your communication, but it can trip you up because of one of those pesky no-talk rules: If you have to talk about sex, then you must not be compatible/passionate enough/sexually skilled. This rule insists: If you have to talk about it, then you are demystifying it, and mystery is the only way to feel erotic!

Fortunately, having some frank and open conversations about sexuality is not a danger to the mystery of sex—sexuality and eroticism are complex, enormous, and powerful areas of human experience. Your conversations will not change that, but they might open up space for honesty and fulfillment that was not there before.

Putting a priority on your sexual relationship also means allotting time for erotic activity. We can schedule every other activity, like time with friends, time with children, time for household chores, not realizing that we haven't allowed time to connect physically and emotionally with our partner. For many people, being sensual and sexual requires genuine relaxation. If you're not rested, it's hard to feel playful. Pressure to perform, to squeeze sex into the last thirty minutes of your day, isn't conducive to pleasure.

If you are currently not partnered and are seeking to feel more sexually inspired, ask yourself some questions. Are any unresolved feelings, especially anger or grief, affecting your sexuality? Are you feeling well, getting rest, nourishing yourself, and moving your body regularly? How do you feel in your body? What do you do to feel sexually attractive? Do you have time to cultivate a sexual connection with someone? Are you involved in activities that will put you in contact with potential partners? As you move through the following chapters, give yourself the gift of taking your time with the exercises.

While pleasure itself may come from something simple, the practice of seeking and feeling pleasure is anything but. Many of us are afraid to feel, period. We hope to feel pleasure without having to feel our other, scarier feelings. That, of course, is not possible in recovery, where we are making room for our discomfort and caring for all the parts of ourselves. Pleasure emerges as we become more enlivened, and we feel more alive as we become freer to be ourselves: full of feelings, memories, hopes, dreams, and living in our bodies as they are, right now.

Sober and Sexual Without Fear

Being sexual without the aid of alcohol or drugs is a huge concern for many in recovery. Some women have difficulty remembering the last time they were sober while having sex, and some have never had sex sober. In addition, many people had unfulfilling and dissatisfying sexual experiences when they did have them while sober.

It was this understanding that started turning the tide toward recovery for Michelle. When she finally confided in a girlfriend that Chris was "trying to control" her drinking, the girlfriend asked whether Michelle had been sober while having sex with him recently. Michelle immediately felt shame, realizing that she couldn't remember the last time she and Chris had been sexual without alcohol. It must have been years ago. Michelle's friend was kind, but she knew that Michelle's drinking was causing harm, and so she asked a question that helped Michelle reflect on her own behavior. Michelle remembered the therapist's office and how difficult it had been to answer questions about their sexual connection.

"We haven't really been having sex at all," Michelle said to her friend. "Not sober, not drunk, for a long, long time." She began to cry as the realization of how lonely and isolated she felt overcame her in big waves. Michelle was terrified of changing her behavior, but deep down she knew her marriage couldn't survive if she didn't. "What do I do?" she asked her friend. "I don't know how to fix this." Her friend encouraged her to take things one day at a time.

"Today," her friend suggested, "tell him how you feel about this. Maybe start reducing the amount of alcohol you're drinking by a third, or by half, just to see how your body responds. Try that for a few days, then maybe try going to a meeting?"

"I can't do AA," Michelle said immediately. "My dad did it every time he got sober, and it never worked." Michelle's friend encouraged her to spend just a few minutes looking for other options, other types of mutual support groups, that might help her. Michelle didn't want to go to a group. She felt sure she could quit drinking on her own, if Chris supported her.

"I'll tell him I'm taking a month off," she decided.

Later that evening, Michelle approached Chris for a conversation. She told him she'd been thinking that she'd like to reduce her drinking, and she was going to try a dry month. She hoped this would motivate him to hold her, kiss her, offer her some affection.

Their therapist had encouraged them to offer each other affectionate touch, and he was able to reach for her in support and gratitude when she told him she was ready to change her habits with alcohol.

Within minutes, when Michelle realized that Chris might want to transition from affectionate touch to sex, she froze. Frustrated with her own body's responses to what should have been a perfect moment to have sex, Michelle ignored the discomfort. Their sex was familiar, but not satisfying for her. Silently, she became afraid that as a sober person, she would have dissatisfying sex for the rest of her life.

Michelle and Chris continued to go to couple's therapy, where Michelle was finally able to speak about her use of alcohol, anxiety medication, and sleeping pills. She told the therapist that she had reduced her drinking and was going to do a whole dry month.

But then, Michelle was unable to go one month without alcohol. The therapist referred her to multiple recovery groups that were based in some ways on AA but had their own style and content.

With support from Chris, Michelle began going to a women's online meeting that felt safe and supportive. She listened to other women discuss their experiences, and eventually, she introduced herself to the group. The word *alcoholic* made her squirm because of how much she associated it with her father, but this group didn't require people to say it. She asked for a sponsor, someone who had been married a long time, had raised children, and could help her navigate some issues in her relationship that needed to be untangled from her drinking.

In couple's therapy, Michelle began to understand that sexual responses are learned responses. Facing the fact that she was frightened to have sexual experiences sober was actually her first step in learning how to have more satisfying sex. Chris and Michelle began to discuss their relationship history openly with the therapist and started to discover more about what the other had been feeling, wanting, and fearing for the past several years.

A Safe Environment
If sex is already frightening because you are going to engage in it sober, then it is crucial to reduce your other anxieties about sex. Start by trying to figure out what makes a sexual experience

comforting and secure for you. You may need to know your partner for some time and explore extensive touching before you become more sexual. Or you may want to be sexual only in the bedroom when the children are asleep. You may need to promise yourself that you will never be sexual out of reaction to pressure from your partner.

Being aware of what you need to feel relaxed, now that you are recovering, will help you get in touch with what makes a sexual situation comfortable for you. Give yourself permission to do whatever makes the sexual experience feel as safe as possible.

When Ash entered sobriety most recently, they were surprised at how sensitive they became to the world around them. "I couldn't tolerate loud noises, crowds, any of the things that had been normal to me when I was drunk and high," Ash says. As Ash began working through their traumatic sexual history, they were finally able to recognize how little pleasure they had ever gotten out of sex. They experienced intense emotions: grief, terror, and rage. They missed their partner, Ben, every day but didn't reach out because they felt too overwhelmed by what they were experiencing.

"This time around," Ash says, "I feel like it's all just here in front of me whether I want to deal with it or not. Like, I have to make a massive change or I'll die, and that's not an exaggeration. I can't survive what I was doing before. If I ever have sex again, I'll probably have to take seven hours just to get naked!"

The Courage to Relearn

If being sexual while sober is new for you, it makes sense for it to bring you some anxiety—most of us have some difficulty trying new things, especially as adults who expect ourselves to be perfect. Your anxiety about sober sex should decrease with experience over time. As your body begins to give you clear feed-back, you will start to become aware of your sexual responses and be better able to predict them. You will learn what pleases you, what feels good, and what you want more of. You will, in many ways, relearn how to have sex.

One night after Michelle had stopped drinking, she was very agitated. She no longer knew how to fall asleep on her own. As she lay awake reading, waiting for Chris to come home, she grew angrier and angrier. *At least if he were here, we could try to have sex,* she thought, *and then I could get some sleep.*

The longer she waited, the more she thought how nice that would be. And then she realized that beneath her feelings of ag-itation, she actually did want to have sex. *Chris may not be home,* she mused, *but I am.* And suddenly masturbation seemed like a great idea. It had been so long since her body had given her the signal of desire that it took her walking through agitation and anger first before she could sense it. She knew that spending some time in her own self-pleasure would feel good, and when Chris got home, he would not feel pressured to "fix" whatever negative feelings she had before.

A Second Adolescence

AA folk wisdom says that you stop growing emotionally when you enter an addiction. On some level, addiction seems to impede sexual development as well as the personal growth process. It's cer-tainly harder to integrate the two while engaged in an addiction.

In recovery, you may feel very young and immature sometimes. You may discover that you feel like a teenager sexually, that you don't really know what you want and you don't know what kind of touch feels most arousing, even if you have already had years of sexual experiences. You may feel that you need to experiment sexually in terms of both techniques and partners. And you can!

However, it is important to proceed with self-awareness, honesty, and consent of all parties, and to stay grounded in your desire to experiment and grow. Many people in early recovery act out sexually in ways they never did when they were addicted, and then they must recover from that behavior too.

If you started drinking or using your substances during adolescence, you never had a chance to get to know yourself sexually; your sexual responses were often filtered through the substances you were using. If you withdrew from sexuality after a traumatic experience, you may feel similarly. Now you may need to go through that period of sexual development and experimentation as an adult. You may feel ashamed and embarrassed to find yourself acting like a teenager, and you may also feel cheated and angry that you have to go through sexual self-discovery as an adult. You are definitely not alone, no matter how you feel about this.

It's never too late to connect with yourself. Allow yourself to feel your feelings and to be exactly where you are in the process. Comfort yourself with the fact that no matter your past, you can do what you need to do to feel safe as you explore your own sexual growth, here today.

○ ◎ ○

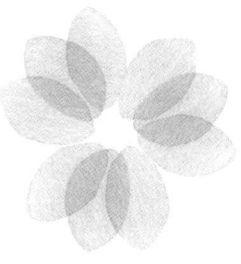

CHAPTER 4

Accepting Your Body

A PRAYER OF GRATITUDE AND COMMITMENT

Dear body, thank you for being in witness to my life. For your unwavering accompaniment. For the blessing you have offered by keeping me alive, keeping me here on earth, so that I may do the work we came to do. I have faith in our partnership, in our ability to be in right relationship both with each other and with the world around us. I commit to acknowledging and honoring your wisdom, to knowing you better each day. I acknowledge your hurt and pain, so that you no longer need to numb, and I invite our community to hold us, so that we may grieve together.

You are my best friend and I am yours.

You are my best friend and I am yours.

You are my best friend. And I am yours.

———

Meenadchi, *Decolonizing Nonviolent Communication*, 2nd ed.

If you've spent any time at a school, at a swimming pool, or walking in a city, you have probably seen many kinds of bodies. It is important for us to appreciate the infinite variety in human bodies, and many of us are happy to join the movement for body positivity—as long as we are talking about somebody else's body. When it comes to our own body, we are usually less accepting. We know exactly what our "bad" points are, and we figure everyone else does too.

In our work with clients, we have found that most people are chronically dissatisfied with their bodies and criticize them constantly. They say things like, "My stomach is too flabby," "My breasts are too saggy," "I'm too old for that," or "Maybe if I were ten pounds lighter . . ."

It is not an overstatement to say it has been normalized for everyone to dislike some part of their body. Negative feelings about our bodies reflect our culture's emphasis on the importance of appearance, especially for women who seek to embody a feminine ideal. Despite many years of feminist activity addressing "beauty culture," privilege still accrues to white, slim, smooth, hair-free, unwrinkled, airbrushed young women, with curves permitted only in a few key places. (At the same time, these very women often report negative feelings about their bodies!)

Sonya Renee Taylor, an activist for radical body acceptance and author of *The Body Is Not an Apology: The Power of Radical Self-Love*, puts it this way: "When our personal value is dependent on the lesser value of other bodies, radical self-love is unachievable."[1] Taylor makes the point that our dissatisfaction with our own bodies is propped up by enormous business interests that profit from our self-hatred. In addition, we perpetuate a culture of prejudice by internalizing messages about size, skin color, ability, age, illness, and which bodies are "better" than others.

Comparing ourselves to a body that seems more valuable sets us up to feel inadequate and less lovable. Likewise, feeling better about our bodies because we are achieving "perfection" (measured against others' imperfect bodies) is not the same thing as true self-acceptance.

Increased access to plastic surgery and cosmetic injectables like Botox is a double-edged sword for us. On the one hand, more people are able to receive gender-affirming care and to live more authentically in their bodies via procedures that were extremely difficult or impossible to obtain thirty years ago. Access to products and treatments that increase confidence and self-regard is a good thing. On the other hand, high-cost procedures are the latest way that many people express their insecurity and stay in a cycle of never-quite-perfect-enough.

Negative messages about our bodies come from many sources. We hear them at home, at school, at work, in our media, in advertisements, and, eventually, inside our own minds. One of the most common negative messages is about body size. Anti-fat bias is a huge source of harm for people in larger bodies and contributes to all our body shame. Americans spend more than

$30 billion on diet products annually, and around 45 million people diet every year.[2]

People seek to be thinner for many reasons. Certainly the privilege that thinner people enjoy extends into many areas of life, including earning more money, finding clothes that fit off the rack, feeling welcome in public spaces, having easier access to competent health care, and so on. It is an unfairness that is baked into our current social world, connected to white privilege, cisgender privilege, male privilege, and class privilege.

No one is immune to the influence of negative messages about body size or shape. The larger someone's body is, the more intense the external social pressure to make their body smaller, no matter the cost to their health or well-being. And body size is only one aspect of our physical existence.

Women receive negative messages about skin color, facial features, hairstyle, dental work, wearing glasses . . . the list goes on and on. For many of us, how we look seems more important to the world around us than how we feel or who we are. It is difficult to feel good, difficult to access pleasure, when you are constantly made to feel bad about your body.

Recent research shows that medical prejudice has caused harm to women and nonbinary, queer, and trans people through a lack of research on women's health and a lack of priority given to women and queer people's experience. There are countless examples: Perhaps most glaring among them is the fact that the rate of maternal mortality in the United States is ten times that of any other developed country. A large racial disparity also exists, with Black women dying at rates over twice that of white women. When queer people who give birth are asked to describe their overall childbirth experience, they describe the impacts of bias and discrimination at significantly higher rates than cisgender, heterosexual people.[3]

Another example is prescription medication. We are only just beginning to understand how gender differences might matter in prescribing drugs to women. Women and gender-diverse people have been taking dosages of many drugs that were tested only on cisgender men "of normal weight." Medical researchers were not required by law to include women in early clinical trials of new drugs until 1993. This means we are still years away from comprehensive, evidence-based, wholistic care for any of us.

Consider that the full shape and scope of the clitoris wasn't known or described until 2005, in a paper by Australian urologist Helen O'Connell. Anyone who received their sexual education before 2005 is now working from an outdated understanding of female anatomy. (It's worth doing a quick search for "anatomical illustration of the full clitoris" to get up to date.)

In addition to a lack of information, we have the harms of systemic racism, homophobia, transphobia, prejudice against disabled and larger bodies—these all add up to serious difficulty for many people when it comes to accessing medical care for the bodies we are already taught to feel shame about. At the same time, doctors are still presumed to be the authorities on our bodies. In short, mainstream American culture has put up extreme barriers to women and gender-expansive people knowing, understanding, and enjoying our own bodies.

The most basic means for knowing anything, especially ourselves, is to touch. Touching ourselves, especially feeling around "down there," has been discouraged for many of us for as long as we can remember. While some, likely younger, women and gender-expansive people may have received more sex-positive messages at home or in the media, the force of shame at school, in extended family, at places of worship, and so on, cannot be overstated.

Our sex-negative culture attaches shame to sexual curiosity while our sex-obsessed culture simultaneously attaches shame to sex avoidance. We live in constant contradictions about how sexual our bodies are supposed to be. We can begin to find calm in the chaos by reconnecting with how our bodies actually feel, right here, right now.

Every person has some sense of their physical being and image. Self-acceptance at any level depends in part on accepting our body as it is, even if we want to make changes. Admiring it and reveling in what it can do rather than focusing on its shortcomings or perceived flaws comes on the heels of this acceptance; it may happen more quickly for some of us than for others, depending on our unique combination of experiences and identities.

If we want to reconnect with the person we are internally, we can't reject bits and pieces as "not okay"; we need to begin to accept every part of us. Our bodies are incredible vehicles and can be miracles of movement and pleasure. We need to accept our bodies as inextricable parts of ourselves and know that all bodies are deserving of care and love. Getting to know your body is the key to unlocking many other doors.

Our body image has a tremendous impact on the quality of our sexuality. Deep down inside you may suspect your partner of cataloging your body's faults. If you view yourself as unattractive, you will be much more likely to want to have sex intoxicated, late at night, in the dark, and hidden under the covers. Feeling flawed on the outside leads to feeling undesirable on the inside. We resign ourselves to living lives of longing because we secretly fear that we are undesirable to others.

The feeling of being undesirable—and thus, undesired—can gradually change. Throughout this chapter, you will have opportunities to initiate change as we learn to adjust the messages we give to ourselves and begin to believe we are all desirable in our unique way. It isn't something we need to earn; it doesn't accumulate partner by partner. Our desire and desirability are part of who we are and what we bring to any sexual relationship.

Making Peace with Your Body

While experiencing a substance use disorder, many people neglect, ignore, or cover up their bodies. A few focus on keeping their bodies "perfect" to hide their addiction. Some women are very focused on their bodies and keep themselves looking a certain way not from a sense of loving their bodies or caring about themselves, but to attract partners or maintain a social image of themselves. An image of perfection and the feeling of being in control can be the goals for compulsive behavior with exercise or the driving impulse for eating disorders. If life feels out of control due to addiction, food restriction or other disordered eating behaviors can seem like a way to regain control.

Others find that trauma leads them to dissociate from their bodies, ignore their body's basic needs, and give up attending to their own health. Both perfectionism and dissociation can lead to more self-harming behaviors.

Recovering people need to acknowledge how they feel about their bodies; they need to look at them and decide to accept them, to care for them, and to listen to them. If you still want to make changes to your body, you can find pathways that are supportive of your overall health.

Let's look through the eyes of women at different stages of recovery to see how body image is an issue in their lives: Tamara, who feels disconnected from her own body due to disability and chronic pain, heavy use of opioid painkillers, grief about her divorce, and the symptoms of menopause; Miyu, who has spent much of her young life either actively anorexic or in recovery from her illness and is just beginning to notice her own sexuality; and Arati, a single mother who struggles with her body image under her own perfectionism and internalized shame.

Tamara

Tamara sat in her mother's hospital room, staring out the window. It was just after eight in the morning, and her heart was still pounding from adrenaline. Her mother, Anne, was getting X-rays in another room, and this was the first moment Tamara had to catch her breath after waking up to the horrible scene in the bathroom. Her mind kept whizzing back to the moment she found Anne moaning in pain on the floor, and then the overwhelming chaos of emergency medical personnel, a stretcher, an ambulance. Tamara pulled off her sweater and fanned herself with her hands. She was burning up. She was nauseated. She wanted to take a pill.

After Tamara's mother had her traumatic fall in the bathroom and fractured her hip, Tamara was overwhelmed with guilt for her own increased use of pain medication. Tamara was certain her mother would not have been as severely injured if Tamara hadn't been sedated by a combination of pills—some prescribed to her, some not. Tamara had been working with a therapist to manage stress and grief, and the therapist recommended a pain specialist who might be able to taper her off opioids and use other medications and methods to manage her pain.

Tamara made a big decision and took a medical leave of absence from her university. She was determined to "handle" her dependency on pain medication. She devoted herself to the plan made by a new pain doctor, continued to see her therapist, and started receiving acupuncture. She researched caregiving support programs and was able to arrange for lower-cost in-home respite care for her mother. This gave Tamara some room to focus more on herself.

All this focus on tapering off pain pills and developing other pain management strategies was very helpful to Tamara, although she still had chronic pain. Eventually, she had to face that her mood was still depressed. She resisted going to a support group for people with opioid use disorder—her university town was small, and she didn't want to risk the stigma of people in the community knowing she was struggling. She resisted joining support groups for people with chronic pain and disability—she presumed they would make her feel sadder. She was sure that following what her new doctor told her to do would change everything, and she would feel good again, all on her own.

Her therapist reflected to her: "It seems like you are trying to fix something about your body that feels wrong to you. Maybe in your thoughts you are comparing yourself to an ideal and finding yourself lacking?"

"I'm comparing myself to a person who isn't dependent on OxyContin and can walk on her own two feet," Tamara snapped back. "That's not much of an ideal."

But the conversation stuck with Tamara. She would never speak that way about anyone else who had chronic pain, or used a cane, and she knew it. She felt betrayed by her body. She felt trapped in her pain, even as she was managing it differently than before. Her body felt uncomfortable, difficult to move, and unattractive. It had been a long time since she felt like she looked good. She suddenly felt angry at Alisha, her ex-wife, for abandoning her. *If Alisha hadn't left, maybe I'd still feel like a woman and not a collection of diseases,* she thought.

A small, wise voice inside Tamara said: *This isn't Alisha's fault. And it's not your body's fault, or your mother's fault, or even really your fault. At the same time, it is up to you to take care of yourself.* Tamara felt a softening inside. She felt that underneath her anger, guilt, and fear, she was very, very sad. And she realized that quitting opioids alone was not going to make her well.

Miyu

Miyu looked down at her thighs, where thin scars crisscrossed in a star pattern. It had been three years since she actively self-harmed with a razor or needed hospitalization for her anorexia, but she wasn't quite ready to show her body, even though it was hot out. She put on long pants and left for therapy.

Miyu had recently started dating a new person, a young man she met at the gym. She had been able to postpone any sexual touch by structuring the dates so that they would be in groups of friends or out during the day. But she knew there would come a time when he would want to kiss her, and she was feeling anxious. When she imagined him seeing her scars, or how her body looked without clothes, she wanted to throw up. She took a deep breath and let it out slowly.

Her therapist asked whether Miyu wanted to kiss this new guy, and she had difficulty coming up with an answer. She settled on "Maybe?" As she said it, she thought about what a statement like that could mean about her. Why didn't she know if she wanted to kiss him?

At twenty-four, Miyu had been in and out of recovery for almost ten years for anorexia and self-harm. She had been to inpatient treatment, intensive outpatient treatment, groups, camps, and now individual therapy to maintain the stability she has worked hard to achieve. Miyu still struggles to eat when she is stressed, but she has a good support system in her family, friends, and therapy, and she has many tools to help herself. She almost never feels the impulse to cut her skin anymore, and she is proud of going three years without using cutting or deliberate food restriction to cope.

Miyu's parents were initially shocked at how sick Miyu had become as a teenager—they did not talk about emotions in their home and were unaware that she was struggling, because she had been able to maintain good grades and never skipped school. Miyu had two siblings, a sister and a brother, who were older and high achievers. The family had been focused on getting them through their stressful period of college applications.

Miyu had been able to hide her skin cutting and food restriction from her family by wearing baggy clothes. She would blame her period when she was nauseated or experiencing abdominal pain from undereating, and push food around her plate while lying about other meals she'd eaten that day. Miyu kept a detailed diary of the calories she consumed and the hours she worked out. Her period had never stabilized, so she did not notice going months without it. She simply wanted to be smaller, which to her meant sexier, ready to be noticed by a man who would scoop her up in his arms. This dream occupied all her attention. She drew pictures of her perfect boyfriend, based on one or two boys at school, or her favorite K-pop star.

Then her grades began to slip, and she fainted at school more than once. The school nurse told Miyu's parents that she might have an eating disorder, and she needed to see a doctor. Miyu did not want to go to treatment, but because she was a minor, she had no choice. She refused to participate in group and was noncompliant throughout most of her first stay in inpatient treatment. She missed much of her senior year of high school. She went back to school, relapsed, went back to treatment, and resisted. Miyu still wanted to be thinner. She completed her General Educational Development (GED) exam while in treatment "because I was bored."

Miyu's parents were stiff and careful in family therapy, but they genuinely wanted Miyu to be well and happy, so they complied with whatever Miyu's doctors suggested. It was a bumpy road. Over the course of a few years, Miyu gradually came to see that her anorexia was causing her real harm, and she started participating in her own treatment. After she turned eighteen, she stayed at home, and her parents helped her navigate the medical and mental health systems she relied on for support.

Now, Miyu has finally moved into an apartment with a friend, has kept a job at a retail store for two years and has been promoted to assistant manager, and is feeling ready to start looking for a relationship. When Jake, the nice-looking guy at the gym, asked for her number, she was relieved! She immediately deleted all the dating apps she had been looking at and started fantasizing about marrying Jake and having a family.

Of course, she'd first have to be able to get over feeling terror about kissing him.

Arati

Running after the bus, juggling her work bag and travel mug, Arati feels a familiar pang of shame. She is going to be late for class again. As a graduate student studying statistics, Arati struggles to maintain her demanding schedule and care for her three-year-old son. She always feels that she is behind the curve, never quite good enough.

Arati became pregnant in college, unmarried and without intention to be a parent at that time. Her parents were horrified that she decided to have a baby without marrying the father, but Arati felt certain, deep down, that this was right for her. Her son's father maintains his financial commitments and sees their child occasionally, but Arati was aware that she was choosing single parenthood when she opted to carry her pregnancy to term.

From the day she was born, Arati's parents had expected their eldest daughter to become a doctor. They had immigrated from India in the 1970s and prioritized creating a path for baby Arati and eventually her two younger sisters to succeed. Since getting pregnant, Arati has felt herself shrink from their judgment and strive to be the best mother and student she can be, even though she is not following their dream for her. Quietly, she knows there is a part of her they will never understand: her sexuality. Arati is attracted to people of all genders and identifies as bisexual. The dissonance she feels inside is sometimes unbearable. She has relied on her parents for financial support and childcare, but she keeps an important part of herself from them.

Without a formal diagnosis of attention-deficit/hyperactivity disorder (ADHD), which would indicate a need for treatment, Arati has become reliant on Adderall, a commonly prescribed stimulant, for energy and concentration. She buys it from a classmate, which is easy and normalized on campus. The Adderall feels necessary on days like today, when she will be on campus for at least ten hours. At night, Arati drinks wine to relax—sometimes half a bottle, usually more.

Recently, Arati met an attractive person at a meetup for LGBTQ+ students in STEM. The new person uses she/they pronouns, flirted easily, and seemed excited to get to know Arati. The two of them exchanged numbers, texted for a few days, and decided to set up a date.

As Arati started getting ready for her date and getting her son ready to go to his grandparents' house, she caught herself in the mirror. She panicked. She realized that even with her years of sexual experience, she felt awkward, unsexy, and disconnected from her own body. She tried to fix her posture, suck in her belly, and roll her shoulders back. It made no difference. She spent a long time picking out clothes that hid most of her body, feeling critical and despairing the whole time.

She also felt guilty for going on a date instead of spending the evening with her son. Arati took extra Adderall, which made her feel slightly nauseated, so she skipped most of dinner. Then, she drank more alcohol than usual, to calm her anxieties.

Arati enjoyed the new person but felt out of control. She knew she was using more Adderall and alcohol than she used to, and it was happening more often. She felt afraid of what might happen if she didn't take action. When she said goodnight to her date, she pushed their hands away from her waist, ashamed of the softness of her body.

Arati took advantage of her campus counseling center and found a queer-friendly therapist who could hold space for her many identities and concerns. The therapist suggested that Arati consider reducing her intake of stimulants and make some time in her busy schedule for self-pleasure and reacquainting herself with her own body. For Arati, neither suggestion sounded easy, but they both sounded right.

Listening to Your Body's Messages

Let's begin with some expectation setting: You may never fall in love totally with how your body looks. The critical external messaging, the pressure to conform to beauty standards, and the way our privilege and marginalizations interplay in and on each person's body—it is a lot to navigate. However, this doesn't mean you are doomed to hatred of your body. In fact, we believe that you can live in a deeper state of acceptance, even gratitude, for your body, exactly as it is right now. And this sets the stage for feeling more sensual, confident, and sexy in your body too. Feeling good about how you look becomes a gift, a lovely addition to a day, but it is no longer the whole goal.

The key to a more neutral, even positive regard for your body is conscious effort toward becoming more aware of how your body feels and what it can do, rather than how it looks or what it can't do. When you listen to your body's messages, you begin to work with rather than against yourself.

We won't pretend that your relationship to your body exists in a vacuum—in fact, most of the negative things you say to yourself are the result of violently cruel biases that you did not invent. The systems that enact body-based oppression won't be changed overnight. We are more able to change systems when we cultivate at least a neutral relationship with our own bodies and positive regard for the bodies of others.

As Jessi Kneeland writes in *Body Neutral: A Revolutionary Guide to Overcoming Body Image Issues*, "Instead of asking people to 'rise above' or 'cast off' their social context, body neutrality asks us to accept, acknowledge, consider, and explore it with open eyes and a clear mind. Only by doing so can we fully recognize the truth that an individual's body is never the actual problem."[4]

Here are a few practical techniques for making better friends with your body. It is safe to cultivate daily awareness of your relationship with your body, feel your body's sensations, and see what your body looks like. If you are used to a lot of negative internal chatter when looking in the mirror, the following exercise is for you.

EXERCISE

The Mirror, Part 1

Find a time when you are alone and undisturbed. Take everything off and stand naked in front of a full-length mirror. If you don't have a full-length mirror, you can do this exercise with a hand mirror, moving it slowly around your body so you can see each part, one at a time. You don't need to prepare your body for this activity—you get to have hair, odor, pimples, dry skin. Let your body exist however it does, right in this moment.

If you find the idea of looking at yourself naked a bit scary, you're not alone. Many people find it difficult to look at their bodies without the camouflage of clothes. The point of this exercise is just to look, not to evaluate. Avoid weighing yourself before or after this exercise; avoid trying to make your body look "better" in the mirror. See if you can look at your body with new eyes—eyes that appreciate your aliveness.

If you have an onrush of negative thoughts, it is time to pause. Write them down, share them with a group or therapist, do a ritual to move them out of your mind. Right now, all you are doing is looking at your own body with soft curiosity. What do you see?

Arati's therapist suggested that she try this exercise. As Arati gazed at herself, she noticed just how many negative thoughts she had about her body. It made her so sad and anxious, she had to stop and get dressed.

When she described her experience to her therapist, she was gently reminded to start slowly and be easy with herself, beginning with one part of her body at a time and extending that area a little bit each day. As she followed her therapist's suggestion, Arati felt considerably less threatened. After several weeks she was able to look at her body in the mirror without the sadness. She recognized it; she found that it could look different depending on the light, the shadows, and how she stood. Most importantly, she began to connect how she viewed her body with what she was already thinking about or what she was feeling that day.

This was a revelation, a real breakthrough in understanding. Arati's body—and how it looked to her—did have a relationship to the "rest" of Arati. They were irrevocably connected. For example, if Arati was stressed about her schoolwork, she felt more critical, usually of her stomach. If she was feeling calm and enjoying affection with her son, she could see her stomach as a hardworking, truly incredible part of her body.

EXERCISE

The Mirror, Part 2

Try simply looking at your body a few times, or for a few weeks. If this causes you significant distress, please back off and get some support. This exercise can be challenging, but it shouldn't send you into a panic. If looking at your body makes you feel panicked or disgusted, it's time to seek some more support.

When you have been able to look at your body without concentrating on some alleged imperfection, you are ready for the next step: to begin to accept your body. Once you have some idea of how you look, see what happens when you deliberately replace any negative appraisal with words of acceptance.

Take a calm, smooth breath. Say aloud to your reflection in the mirror, "You're fine. I like you just the way you are. This is okay. This body is okay." Even if you don't fully believe this statement, saying it aloud opens the possibility that it could be true, and that's the beginning of the change we seek. Research on affirmations consistently supports the idea that even when we don't totally believe them, saying positive words to ourselves aloud helps us maintain a more positive self-view.

Now the real challenge: Go slowly over your body, expressing love to every part, as you would to the body of a beloved child. First do it verbally: Thank your body for being there, express appreciation for what it does for you. For example, you may thank your feet for helping you to walk and run and dance. You may thank your neck for allowing you to look behind you. You may thank your spine for allowing you to bend over. You may thank your shoulders for carrying your bags around. No matter how awkward you might feel, see if you can take a full tour, saying something kind and expressing some gratitude toward every part of you. Once you have done it, sit quietly for a minute and see how you feel. Listen to your body.

Arati was able to do this portion of the exercise for only a few moments before she felt overwhelmed. She felt silly, and she found it almost unbearable. She realized she had no problem doing something similar for her own son—she often played with him by telling him she loved his arms, legs, belly, feet. Why was it so difficult to do it for herself? She didn't know, but she was determined to keep trying. As she kept practicing over the passing weeks, her embarrassment faded away, and she came to look forward to her time with herself. The discomfort of really being with herself gave way to anticipation of this new ritual she had claimed for herself.

One day Arati's therapist mentioned that Arati's presence had changed. She seemed calmer, warmer. Arati smiled, because she could feel it too. "I feel my butt in the chair in class," she said. "I feel the air on my skin outside. When I kiss my son, I can really smell him and feel his skin. Being a grad student feels like I'm supposed to live only in my head. The rest of my body is just there to keep my brain going. I'm tired of that. I want to feel my whole body again."

Listening to our bodies is a difficult task for most of us. We expect our bodies to simply function exactly as they always have, regardless of how much care we are offering. On days when you don't feel friendly with your body, it is important to remind yourself that your feelings are an understandable response to the relentless negative messaging from our family, community, culture, and media.

Many of us have spent years emotionally disconnected from our bodies. We are not encouraged to do otherwise. Learning to befriend your body is a progression over time. For those who are experiencing pregnancy, gender transition, healing from a surgery, or any other major change to the body, this activity can be both especially challenging and especially supportive. However you feel about your body's changes, both your feelings and your body are okay.

After you can really look at your whole self naked in the mirror for the first time without dismay and disappointment, you may gradually feel a sense of familiarity and tolerance, maybe even reassurance. Finally, the acceptance of and care for your body as you now know it will develop. This is a major step toward sexual recovery, one that you have made happen.

Many of us are not able to accept our bodies overnight, but eventually, with practice, we will begin to appreciate and even enjoy our uniqueness. Even if you still want to make changes to your body, you can decide to accept your body in the present, feel okay about it, and be grateful, knowing it is precious just the way it is.

EXERCISE

Listening Without Looking

Lie down and close your eyes, and begin to feel what's happening inside of you. Feel your breath moving in and out. Feel how it fills your lungs and empties out again. Feel your chest rising and falling. Feel the beat of your heart. Listen for the sound it makes as it pumps blood throughout your body. Feel your blood circulating to every part of you, keeping you alive. Give your body your appreciation for doing this all by itself, without needing any help at all from your conscious mind.

What About Your Genitals?

While we will be focusing on the experience of people with vulvas in this section, it is important to remember that the experience of being a woman is not dependent upon being born with female anatomy, and there are plenty of people born with vulvas who go on to live as trans men or have more complex gender identities.

For nonbinary or intersex people who want to avoid the language of female anatomy, there are a few gender-neutral terms that often circulate: *bits*, *parts*, *privates*. Intersex people, often born with atypical genitals, are nearly always assigned a binary sex identity by their doctors or parents—a practice many people are working to change. Some trans people adopt terms for their genitals that are in line with their gender identity; others may not. While many trans women opt for gender-affirming surgeries, many do not, or cannot afford to. The true diversity and variety of human genitals is not reflected in our society's current language or practices. The terminology we use for our genitals is both deeply personal and a reflection of our culture.

If we don't know what our genitals look like or what to call them, and the very thought of them makes us blush, it is not surprising that we have a difficult time enjoying ourselves as sexual creatures. "Touch me here; don't touch me there" may be about as specific as we can get. And if we don't want to or cannot look at ourselves, we're not going to be fully comfortable with a lover looking at us. Nor is it easy to seek out or create spaces where we feel sexual all by ourselves.

Many women have never looked at their own genitals. As young children, curious about their genitals as they are about other parts of their bodies, some may have done some self-exploration. Yet frequently we learn early in life that this is not permissible, and so we don't do it, or we feel guilty when we do. Add in the messages we hear from advertisers: that we need a douche or deodorant spray and that panty liners keep us "fresh," and it makes sense why so many women become discouraged from exploring their own genitals. Period-care companies are still unable to use "realistic" blood-like substances in advertisements, because it would be too upsetting.

Another contributor to the difficulty people have in talking about their own genitals is that access to comprehensive sexuality education in public schools is not consistent across the country. While most young people have internet access, they may not have trusted adults who are both compassionate and well informed. Increasingly, young people receive messages about their bodies through exposure to pornography. But pornography is designed to entertain and titillate, not to educate or inform.

In advice forums across the country, it is still common to hear concerns from young women who are disturbed that one of their labia is twice as big as the other. They may be so ashamed of this "defect" that they are anxious about sexual contact with a partner. The fact is most people with vulvas have one shorter and one longer labia minora. It is more common than not.

In all humans, the same variation that occurs among other body parts also occurs among genitals. For example, most people have one foot that is slightly larger than the other, and no one's ears are in perfect symmetry. Some women have breasts of two different cup sizes. Why would our genitals be any different?

A lack of exposure to basic sexuality information can cause deep distress, shame, and negative self-image. It also leads to higher rates of unwanted pregnancies, STIs, and unwanted sexual experiences.

Over the years, many people have tried to counteract these forces. Betty Dodson's *Sex for One: The Joy of Selfloving* (originally published in 1987) included many hand-drawn images of vulvas, illustrating the diversity and variety of normal bodies. More recently, Women's Health Victoria produced *The Labia Library*, a collection of photos that show many types of vulvas. Artist Sam Hil Atalanta created The Vulva Gallery and The Body Diversity Gallery on Instagram, where anyone can see color drawings and paintings of hundreds of people's perfectly normal, different parts. A simple Google search of the question "Are my labia normal?" will return many articles about how when it comes to vulvas, variation is the rule, not the exception.

EXERCISE

Exploring Your Genitals

This exercise has become a popular touchstone for those who are interested in sexuality. You may be tempted to skip it, especially if you have done it a time or two in the past, but we encourage you to make the effort here and now. Doing this exercise as part of your sexual recovery is about becoming the person who knows your body the best.

Do this exercise when you are alone and feel safe and undisturbed. You can approach it with two objectives: to see what's there and to feel what happens when you touch various parts of yourself.

For this exercise, you will need a hand mirror and a flashlight. Sit propped up, maybe with pillows behind your back, and your knees bent and open. You may want to also put pillows under your knees to help you maintain this position comfortably. If it is physically difficult for you to touch your vulva, feel free to use a toy, a partner, or another solution so you can still look and explore.

Begin by looking at your genital area when you're not excited. How many different parts can you see? Can you name them? Do you know what their function is physically and sexually? Are you familiar with your normal aroma, and can you sense when it changes?

Do this exercise once a week for a month. If you have a regular menstrual cycle, see if your genitals change as your cycle progresses. See if it is possible to relax into the exercise and even enjoy your exploration.

When Miyu was tasked with this exercise, she thought it would be easy. She was familiar with the basics of female anatomy. Yet she was genuinely surprised to realize that she had never connected this information with her own body. When she looked into her own vagina, she had the feeling of looking at a completely unknown world.

Miyu looked at herself with utter fascination. She noticed that the outer lips were a pinkish brown and smooth, while the inner lips were nearly purple on the edges and pinker inside.

She felt surprised at how wrinkly her inner labia seemed! As she did this week after week, she noticed that sometimes she was dry and sometimes more lubricated, depending on where she was in her cycle.

It was some time before she was able to touch herself. She was horribly embarrassed, even though she was alone. Miyu had no conscious memory of ever touching herself, except when she washed herself or wiped after urination.

As she began to touch herself, she found herself pulling her finger away instantly. She felt guilt and shame—the remnants of early childhood messages. *Slow down*, she told herself, *slow down. You can do this. It is okay to do this.*

She touched each part gently—her outer lips, inner lips, clitoris, and vaginal opening. She began to ask herself questions: *Is it slippery? No, more like a petal, dry and smooth. Oh, that's kind of bumpy. I wonder if it's always like that.*

When she was able to relax, Miyu began to notice how the rest of her body felt when she touched each area. Each part of her vulva gave her a slightly different and unique sensation.

Giving Yourself Sexual Pleasure

If you had trouble with the last part of that exercise, read on. You'll see that you're not alone.

Most women in recovery, whether from trauma, substance use disorders, eating disorders, or other compulsive behaviors, have spent their whole lives trying to figure out what other people want. The desire to receive caring attention, approval, and validation can drown out any other desire, especially those deemed "selfish."

This socialization undermines our knowledge of ourselves. We may deny we have sexual feelings. We may fake orgasms to please or appease a partner. We may emphasize the physical activity of sex with no connection to our emotional self. We may have no model for growth or understanding.

Just getting a partner to have sex with us is supposed to be enough, but the rest doesn't take care of itself. When we ask ourselves what satisfies us sexually, we genuinely may not know. We may think that our satisfaction is always the result of our partner's satisfaction, or we may realize that we have an old idea of our own sexuality that hasn't grown or changed since we formed it. For some, a lack of sexual pleasure over time is so entrenched, we may feel we need to just give up and "accept" that sexual feelings aren't going to happen. This is different from asexuality—it is numbness.

The ability to give ourselves sexual pleasure is an important part of developing positive feelings about ourselves as sexual beings. We all had different childhood experiences concerning touching ourselves. Miyu, as we have seen, never let her hand stray "down there." Tamara didn't really discover her sexual self until she began dating women in college. Arati had always enjoyed sex and masturbation, but she lost touch with her sexual self after having a baby. Ash knows how to please men, but only as a means to an end. Similarly, Nova can navigate the complex world of eroticism and sexual titillation but has difficulty feeling pleasure for herself. Michelle has felt beholden to her husband, Chris, for sexual satisfaction, only beginning to enjoy masturbation again after working on her sobriety.

Historically, women have received many negative messages about masturbation. Cultural messages about self-pleasure have been changing rapidly, but not in a consistent way. Women, non-binary people, and other gender-expansive people have increased access to gender-affirming sex toys and sex education if they reside in certain states. In other states, however, young people may be told in school that any sexual activity not aimed at reproduction is a sin, or that masturbation is really self-abuse.

Some religions believe that masturbation is a carnal activity that debases your moral character or fiber. Other negative messages can creep into our lives without being stated explicitly, such as: If masturbation is tolerated, it is only for women without partners. It's something you do as a last resort, and even then, it's "abnormal."

In the United States, some people are receiving both types of messages at the same time! Their favorite music may celebrate a wet vagina, while their family shames any expression of sexuality at all. Rather than receiving a clear set of guidelines, most people are existing in a complex set of different, often conflicting values. Vast disparities in sexual education and beliefs about sexuality affect each person's development.

We encourage you to reflect on what messages you have received about your own sexual exploration and what your beliefs and values are now.

We have heard women express the fear that if they masturbate, especially with a vibrator, they won't enjoy partnered sex as much. We maintain that the causes of dissatisfaction when having sex with a partner generally have more to do with the quality of the relationship than with how, or how often, one of the partners masturbates. Vibrators are assistive technology, and none of the research indicates that they cause harm to those who use them.

The reasons to masturbate are powerful: One, it feels good. And two, the more you know about how your body responds, the more you know what you like. This can help you to help your partner give you pleasure, but it is wonderful simply to know yourself. There are other reasons to masturbate: It can provide a good release for vague anxieties, it can help you relax for sleep, it is good for your fantasy life, it is a good way to love yourself, and it is fun to see what happens.

If you have been dependent on alcohol or other substances, you may have had a depressed sexual response and need to learn that you can have a satisfying sexual experience. Women who have been sexually abused may also experience conflict and have difficulty with sexual pleasure and orgasm.

Masturbation is a great way to begin to reconnect with your sexual responses. By stimulating yourself gently and with care, you can learn how you respond to different forms of touch. If you have had abusive sexual experiences, it is very important to be particularly gentle and caring with yourself.

Our advice for all, whether you are new to touching your own body or have years of experience: Go slowly. Use a lubricant on your more sensitive skin. Try several different strokes or pressures. Try a different kind of toy, if you like to use them. If you feel you'd like some more instruction or ideas, and have the financial capacity to pay for access, the library of videos at OMGYES.com is extensive and helpful. You can also check out *Becoming Cliterate* by Laurie Mintz or *Come as You Are* by Emily Nagoski.

You may find the orgasms you have alone are physically more powerful than an orgasm experienced with a partner. This is because no one else knows your body as well as you do, and only you can know what you are feeling from moment to moment. There is no one else's pleasure to think about and distract you. If you don't like what you're feeling, you can stop or change immediately. If you're pressing too hard, you can lighten up. If you need to go more slowly or quickly, you can. And you don't have to waste a moment agonizing over or negotiating how to explain it to your partner. With time and experience, partner sex can become very satisfying, although it will always be different from solo sex.

Perhaps you have the opposite experience and find that only partner sex feels satisfying to you; masturbating isn't appealing to you. There is nothing wrong with preferring partnered sex. However, if you feel dependent upon another person for your pleasure, the relationship can take on addictive qualities. (If this dependency is an agreed-upon type of kink play, known as orgasm denial, then by all means, enjoy!) The point here is that you take the time to get to know your own body's sexual responses and take responsibility for your own pleasure, regardless.

Remember: Orgasm is lovely, but it is not the only type of sexual pleasure you can enjoy. Having the goal of reaching orgasm can put too much pressure on you, create anxiety, and make orgasm more difficult to achieve. Try a looser goal of spending some time feeling good, offering yourself some pleasure without expecting to orgasm. Ironically, these are the conditions under which an orgasm is more likely to arrive!

We will return to masturbation and exploring our bodies later in chapter 10. With a foundation of more friendly acceptance of our bodies, more conscious attention to our senses, and more effort toward sexual pleasure, we can turn our focus in the next chapters to the story of our sexual life until now and what we want for our sexual life going forward.

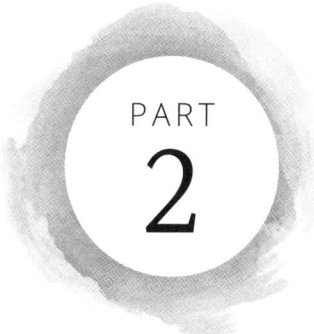

PART

2

Actions: The Outer Journey

Just as the inner journey of early recovery requires us to be honest about our thoughts and feelings, the outer journey requires us to look honestly at the patterns of our behavior. Here we focus on our relationships and sexual interactions. It can be very difficult and painful to acknowledge what has happened and what is happening in our lives today. We need to take this process step by step, recognizing that self-care during this process is recovery in action.

Here are the topics we will address in part 2:

- **Exploring childhood and family sexual issues.** How did your family deal with sexual issues? How did they talk or not talk about sexual issues? What did they call things? How did they explain things?

- **Honestly naming the sexual events of your personal past.** This includes developing your own history and naming the events accurately to your understanding.

- **Looking at your own sexual behaviors,** including charting your sexual and compulsive or addictive behaviors. How did your sexual experience and addictive behaviors influence and interact with one another?

- **Looking at your selection of sexual partners.** Who have you been sexual with and why? What were the characteristics of the relationship?

- **Practicing living in the present.** This is essential to sexuality.

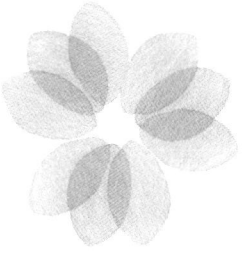

CHAPTER 5

Exploring Sexual Behavior Patterns

*I wish for you a grand and glorious opening—
an unbinding of old fears and judgments,
a softening into sexual joy, curiosity, and
abundance. May you bask in the sun and
welcome light into any hidden places. May
you honor the dark and learn from its
mysteries. May laughter ripple through your
sex play, and may you awaken fully to the
wonder of your own succulent, wild self.*

———

SARK, author of *Succulent Wild Woman: Dancing with Your Wonder-full Self!* 25th Anniversary Edition, personal interview

The outer journey of sexual recovery involves looking at our lives from a fresh perspective. Now the inner work we have done bears real fruit: We can see more clearly and be more honest with ourselves about what we see. Our understanding of our past actions and present interactions continues to deepen as our recovery unfolds. As inauthenticity melts away, we begin to understand the motivations behind our past actions and to see what we can do today to nurture sexual growth and expansion.

Emerging Patterns

Patterns of sexual behavior that you were only dimly aware of in early recovery will now begin to emerge with greater clarity. Looking honestly at your sexual past is essential to sexual recovery. When you can see the patterns in your sexual relationships, you can begin to understand them, and then you can change them if you choose. In recovery there is a link between seeing and understanding who you have been in relationship to others, and growing into who you want to be. Understanding the past is crucial to creating the life you want now and ongoing.

You may find many reasons to avoid looking at your sexual history. Repeatedly, in group counseling and private sessions, at conferences and online, we have heard these reasons for avoidance:

"My old life is over and done with. What's the point of stirring up old memories?"

"My past hasn't affected me. Anyway, I'm starting fresh now."

"I'm clean and sober now, and my past sexual actions were part of my addiction. Why should I look at them? I can't apologize for stuff I don't remember!"

"My life is finally getting stable. Looking at my sexual patterns will just bring on more pain."

"I'm not that person anymore."

We may be very uncomfortable with the idea that our sexual past has the power to affect our present sexual behavior. However, understanding how we've been formed allows us to change. Knowing ourselves and our history opens more future possibility of sexual freedom and choice.

Survivors of sexual trauma may feel they are walking a tightrope at first. Co-author Vanessa remembers the disorienting feeling of balancing a desire to take an honest look at what had happened and how they had acted in response, with a desire to avoid experiencing retraumatization or shame. It is very true that recalling traumatic events without adequate support can be retraumatizing. As you proceed with the self-awareness tasks ahead, we encourage you to choose a pace that is safe for you and to rally the support you need for yourself. This might mean calling a trusted friend, sponsor, or recovery accountability partner, talking about the process in therapy, or calling a support line.

Sometimes you will need a boost of courage to look at the reality of your life. Sometimes you will need permission to go slowly, rest, and recuperate.

Ash had great difficulty accepting that there was a pattern of abuse in their relationships. During their first experience with sobriety, Ash resisted talking about their sexual past. They had taken great pains to construct a self-image of resilience and strength. Although they were aware that they had been sexually abused as a child, they had never considered subsequent sexual experiences as abuse, because they usually were getting basic survival needs met via sex: housing, drugs, physical safety, and so on.

As a young adult, Ash had created a relationship with Ben that was based on mutual respect, but ultimately Ash experienced mental health symptoms and behaviors that made Ben feel unsafe. For Ash, the loss of this relationship was the most pressing issue, not their past. But a small voice within Ash asked for a deeper look at Ash's sexual history, hoping to find clues to the present.

Working with a trauma therapist, Ash found that talking about their sexual patterns brought up painful material that had been buried for many years, including memories of sexual abuse by adults other than their stepfather. "I thought that when I was younger, I was using people to survive," Ash recalled. "But they were abusing me—I was a minor!" This was an important distinction for Ash to make.

At the same time, when Ash reflected on their behavior as an adult, they could see how they had continued a pattern of having sex as a means to an end. "I did end up using some people, and hurting them," Ash said. "And some of them ended up hurting me too." Ash told their therapist about the partner they had before Ben, with whom they had returned to heroin and alcohol time and again. "We had physical fights," Ash remembered. "Getting high and having sex was one of the best ways to end the fighting."

While seeing a trauma therapist, Ash continued to work through the Twelve Steps with their sponsor. Ash had used alcohol and drugs since adolescence to cope with the pain of trauma in their life and to drum up confidence in terrifying situations. Now that Ash was sober, the grief they felt about their sexual relationships was overwhelming. "I don't want to go over every detail of who did what to whom," Ash remembers telling their AA sponsor. "I want to acknowledge that I caused a lot of harm, and that a lot of harm was done to me, and that sometimes those things were happening at the same time. I don't want to make another list of wrongs."

Ash's sponsor saw the wisdom in this choice, even though it went counter to Twelve Step traditions. For Ash, the catalog of abuse and harm was less important than the acknowledgment that they had not always been in control and the reasons why. Ash needed to process their original sense of betrayal and fear stemming from their childhood sexual abuse and abandonment by their mother, and so that was where they put their energy.

While Ash's trauma therapist walked them through their painful memories and experiences slowly—with care and containment using EMDR techniques, journaling, and group support—Ash's AA sponsor kept them accountable to their sobriety. Eventually Ash was able to examine how their life had been patterned off their childhood experiences and see that their sexuality had been bearing a great burden. They felt more tender toward their younger self and cultivated their sense of self-compassion. Ash kept working as a peer mentor at a treatment center, stayed sober, and worked on building more trust in their friendships.

"I'll never not be a survivor," Ash is now able to say. "But I'm not running from my past all the time. It isn't all of who I am."

Acknowledging your sexual history can be emotionally challenging. Your history may not stem from childhood sexual abuse like Ash's did, but everyone has a history that leads us to think, feel, and act the way we do now. Looking at the patterns in your sexual interactions may bring up a multitude of feelings you may not be able to anticipate and don't want to have.

We believe that acknowledging your past, to the extent that you can, will help you move on to a healthier future. It requires a measure of faith in the process and in the resilience of your inner self. The following sections will guide you through acknowledging your past, recognizing patterns, and making clear choices about what you want to bring forward in your life and what you don't.

Childhood and Family Sexual Issues

The first task of the outer journey is to seek out the truth of your early childhood and family sexual experiences. Your sexuality, which includes your most basic ideas of what sex is and what it means, was formed in the crucible of your early childhood experiences. Here you began to absorb the messages about sex that stay with you throughout your life. You can bring those messages out of your unconscious, make them explicit, look at your beliefs about sexuality, and recognize where you got them.

Memories

Begin with your memories. Remember and say aloud or write down what you experienced related to sexuality in childhood. The behaviors and attitudes of your parents, grandparents, aunts and uncles, foster parents, older siblings, and other caregivers have greatly influenced your feelings about your body, your sexuality, and your relationships. Recalling those behaviors and attitudes and being specific about particular incidents will lead to more memories and insights about the connections between your household's attitudes and your own.

If you are not in therapy or in a recovery support group, writing in a personal journal or the *Awaken Your Sexuality Workbook* is a great step toward acknowledging the role sexuality played in your family.

Ask yourself the following questions:

- How did your parents or caregivers express their feelings toward each other? Were they affectionate in front of you? Did a parent or caregiver make jokes about how hard it was to get their partner into bed? Did a parent or caregiver act as if sex were a burden they had to endure?

- Did your parents or caregivers speak openly with you about the changes you would experience in adolescence, or about sexual boundaries, safer sex, or pregnancy prevention?

- Was there ever a conversation about queer sexuality, or were you expected to be heterosexual?

- If you had a complex family system with divorce or multiple parents and stepparents, did you notice a different culture in different households?

- What *didn't* your parents or caregivers say?

- If you had contact with grandparents, did their values seem similar to or different from your parents or caregivers?

Your answers to these sorts of questions will begin to create a richer picture of the messages you received about sex and gender, and how they were conveyed. Now go deeper and explore the emotional tone.

- Were messages about sex expressed as warnings and admonitions, or were they more implicit, contained in silences and holes in the conversation?

- Were your caregivers calm and relaxed about sexuality, perhaps hoping not to create too much tension for you? Remember how you felt during these times.

Investigating these memories may be challenging. If you were sexually abused as a child, or suspect you might have been, individual therapy and maybe other supports are encouraged. You may want to seek out a counselor who is experienced in working with childhood sexual trauma and knows how to help clients recover from childhood abuse, like Ash did.

Some people who experienced childhood abuse are unable to fully recall specific incidents, and that does not mean their pain is less severe. Ash, for example, had clear memories of some of the abuse they experienced from their stepfather, but they also had long stretches of childhood they could not remember at all. Their trauma therapist was able to help them accept this difficult aspect of their trauma.

Trauma affects our memory. Some theorize that this is protective: The less we remember, the less we might suffer it. Others believe that the memories are simply repressed, still residing in the body. Either way, if you are having symptoms in the present, such as recurring nightmares, panic attacks, addictive behaviors, and so on, and you suspect they are connected to childhood sexual abuse or other family violence, finding the right support team is a priority.

Talking with Your Family Members

Talking to your siblings, cousins, or other family members about what they remember experiencing as children can be helpful. You may get validation of your own feelings, and you will certainly get insights into how others in your family remember what happened. You may not recognize the characters in their memories, because their perceptions or experiences were different from yours, which is an important source of information.

Before you approach your family members for this type of conversation, consider whether they are capable of a calm, adult conversation about sexuality. You also need to ask them for their consent to participate. If there was abuse, addiction, or another form of trauma in your childhood, your family members have their own painful memories, and they may not be as ready as you are to discuss them.

If you are in contact with your parents or primary caregivers and feel they can safely discuss these issues with you, a conversation about their values and choices during your childhood may be enlightening. Your parents may find it easier to reveal their discomfort and uneasiness about sex and the way they raised you now that your childhood is over. They may even feel remorseful about their sexual attitudes and how they passed them on. They may welcome the opportunity to express the dissatisfaction they now feel about their own child-rearing practices, and they may share in greater detail how they were raised.

Sometimes the value of talking to a parent is not in getting validation or information, but in the process itself. Being direct, candid, and assertive can be an important personal achievement, regardless of the response. If the idea of talking with your parents about this makes you feel panicked, slow down and investigate the fear. You get to choose how you proceed, as always. This could be challenging, but it shouldn't be an added trauma.

Your goal in talking to your parents or primary caregivers about their sexual attitudes when you were a child is to learn more about the sources of your beliefs about sexuality as an adult. If you enter a conversation with expectations about changing your parents' beliefs, you will probably be disappointed. If you expect an apology for what you regard as their harmful attitudes during your childhood, you probably won't get it. But if you earnestly desire to learn more about the way sexuality was dealt with in your parents' own households growing up, you may come away from the conversation understanding more about your own attitudes and where they come from. The ability to communicate with others about your attitudes is key to your own self-understanding, acceptance, and growth.

For several weeks after a news story broke about a celebrity sexual predator, Michelle's recovery group had been discussing how they learned about sex and boundaries as young people. The news story had triggered painful memories and symptoms for a few women in the group with histories of childhood sexual abuse, and as the group supported them, conversations kept returning to how much each person had been affected in their sexual attitudes and self-understanding by their family of origin.

Many of the women in the group had experienced inappropriate attention from older relatives or family friends, and they discussed how unprepared most of them felt to say no, how difficult it was to tell anyone, and how not being believed had affected them.

Emboldened by the stories of other women in the group, Michelle finally shared with her group that she had been sexually assaulted years before, while working as a young paralegal, and in the outpouring of support she received, she was able to process some of her fear, shame, and rage about the event.

"I feel like I led him on for months," Michelle told the group, "because I didn't want to hurt his feelings. I never said yes anytime he came on to me, but I never really said no." Michelle felt angry at herself now. "I felt like I couldn't move or speak when he attacked me. I didn't even say no then."

A woman in Michelle's group spoke up immediately, saying, "Michelle, he showed you exactly why you were afraid of him— you were trying to stay safe from someone who was crossing boundaries left and right. You may not be the first woman he's hurt, and you're probably not the last. You were trying to avoid making him angry; it makes total sense!"

Another woman chimed in with more support: "You froze. It's totally normal. You didn't say no because you couldn't have. Your brain took over and froze you because you were under threat. You didn't do anything wrong. He never should have put you in a position to say no to him in the first place."

"How did you learn all this?" Michelle asked. The answers were varied. Some women in the group had been educated about sexual boundaries in a more comfortable and mature way, while others, like Michelle, remembered mostly silence and discomfort around the topic from childhood. Some had therapists who had recommended books to them about recovering from sexual abuse, harassment, rape, or violence. Some had met other women in treatment centers or in the criminal legal system who were dealing with the effects of their trauma. A few had partners who had helped them find greater understanding of love and safety.

What they all had in common was that they had to do self-education as adults, as they matured, had new experiences, and developed their own sense of what their sexuality meant to them.

One woman in the group shared that her mother had been raped and had always told her and her sisters that they needed to stick together and "kick him in the shins" if anyone tried to touch them. "She never said anything about how sex might be nice for us," the group participant shared. "It was always about protecting ourselves from men." Michelle realized there was a lot she didn't know about her mother, Donna. She wondered when and how Donna's ideas about sexuality and boundaries had formed.

Michelle had always felt uncomfortable discussing sex with her mother, and she remembered how, when she got her first period, her mother had told her she needed to "lock her knees together." Michelle's father was experiencing active addiction to alcohol throughout all of Michelle's childhood, and Michelle realized she never saw him and Donna expressing playfulness, affection, or attraction to each other.

The women in Michelle's group all agreed to have at least one conversation that week with a person in their life who had affected their understanding of sexuality—for some, whose parents were not alive or safe to contact, this might be another relative or an old friend.

Michelle was surprised that her mother seemed open to having a phone conversation about her sexual attitudes during Michelle's childhood. In fact, when Michelle brought up that she would like to ask some questions about her mother's own upbringing, it seemed almost like Donna had been waiting for permission to share her story.

Donna's parents met in high school, just before Donna's father, Michelle's grandfather, was deployed in the Pacific Theater of World War II. "They never talked about the timing," she said, but it was clear from how quickly they married and had their first son that "they probably got pregnant and had to make that choice." Donna remembered her mother teaching her how to snap together her girdle and cloth menstrual pads, and she also remembered a single conversation about how she should remain "pure" and never let a man put his hands or lips on her until he was her husband.

"Of course I didn't heed that advice," Donna chuckled. Michelle was a little surprised, because she had never imagined her mother having relationships before her father. "I went with a lot of boys before your father," Donna said, "and that was the difference. Your father was a young man."

"So why did you always tell me to wait to have sex until I was married?" Michelle asked.

"Because I didn't always have fun," Donna said quietly. "Being seen as loose in those days meant that some boys thought they could just take what they wanted from you."

Suddenly, Michelle realized her own mother had experienced sexual assault, and they had never talked about it. She felt a wave of grief, and compassion, for the shame her mother seemed to still feel. Michelle took a deep breath and said, "So you thought you were helping me stay safe from dangerous situations by scaring me away from being 'loose.'"

Donna let out a sigh. "I guess so," she said. "Your father didn't care about my past; he just thought I was smart and funny, and we got along so well for the first few years, I always felt I owed him a debt of gratitude."

During that phone call, Michelle had the sensation of fitting puzzle pieces together while her mother continued to talk about her own history. It made more sense to Michelle that Donna had put up with Michelle's father's alcoholism, if Donna felt ashamed of how she had behaved before they were married. It made more sense why they never spoke about sex; it would bring up her own mother's traumatic experiences.

Michelle realized she had been putting a great deal of expectation on herself, and on her husband, Chris, because she wanted to do "better" than her mother had in marriage. She cried after hanging up the phone, and she wrote down some notes about her experience to share back to her group.

Challenges to Healthy Sexual Development in Childhood

Many otherwise constructive, healthy families simply falter when it comes to sex. It is a powerful, difficult issue. Because sexuality is so polarizing in American society and can be so emotionally difficult for parents to discuss, most of us received some form of negative messaging, even if it came in the form of silence.

As younger generations of parents seek to improve on what they experienced as children, there are more resources available to support developmentally appropriate conversations about sexuality and gender. Still, sex educators, medical doctors, psychotherapists, and other workers in sexuality attest to the fact that we have a long road ahead of us.

There are a number of ways families can negatively affect our sexual development, ranging from uncomfortable teasing to the trauma of sexual abuse. Only you know the extent to which your own childhood experiences have affected you, but maybe it will help to read through a list of both more and less common experiences and see if any of them apply to you. We and the women and nonbinary people we have worked with have identified the following challenges:

- My family gave me incomplete and confusing information about sexual development and what I could expect during sexual experiences.

- My parents always told me to cover my body. They didn't want me "offering myself" to boys that way, which made me feel insecure and afraid of male sexuality.

- My mother put me on multiple diets, shaming my body's size and telling me I'd never get a man if I was fat. But I *am* fat and have been my whole life, no matter what I do. It's taken me years of recovery from my eating disorder to allow my body to be the size it actually is.

- I was playing "doctor" with my friend, at a very young age, before I was even aware of sex. My grandmother caught us, sent my friend home, and then locked me in my room for hours. I was ashamed and terrified, and I had no idea what I'd done wrong.

- My religion was very clear: Don't feel sexual desire, and if you do, definitely don't be gay. By twelve, I knew I didn't belong, because I wanted to kiss girls. I had to stay closeted until I was old enough to move out.

- My aunt was always making inappropriate sexual comments to me, talking about my body changing or asking me about my sexual experiences. She would tell me about the men she had sex with, when I didn't want to know!

- A friend of my parents always had excuses to touch me, hugging me or playfully pushing me against the wall and pinning me with his body, and I let it happen, I guess because it would have caused more of a scene if I'd tried to say no.

- My parents had separate beds, separate bed tables, separate lamps. The beds were always perfectly made, as if no one had ever slept in them. I can't imagine how they ever got close enough to one another to conceive me!

- I was sexually abused by my aunt and uncle on and off for years. When I tried to ask my cousins if anything like that had ever happened to them, they yelled at me, called me a liar who would say anything for attention, and cut me off from that side of the family.

- My parents were always talking about their sex life with me and my siblings present. They always said they just wanted us to be informed and comfortable with sex because it was such an important part of life. But the older I got, the more I realized they had never accounted for the possibility that they might be crossing our boundaries.

- I had a teacher who would make me stay after class, alone. He would sit right next to me and lean over me while

I did "extra credit." He was always breathing into my ear, and eventually he touched himself while I kept filling out worksheets. I felt so sick and embarrassed, but I never told anyone.

- When I was leaving for college, my mom asked if I had any questions about sex. We'd never talked about it, and I was already having sex with my boyfriend, so I shrugged her off. She said, "Good, I thought you probably knew everything already." I wonder where she thought I got my information.

These events can have different effects on different people. Rather than define *healthy sexuality* in terms of how bodies should look or behave, we can think of healthy sexual functioning as the consequence of honesty, clear communication, and free choice. Some measure of embarrassment or discomfort during adolescent sexual development is to be expected, but the feeling of being trapped in sexual experiences we do not want is an indication of abuse.

We may discover that we have very different values from our parents, which is common. This is especially true for queer, trans, and nonbinary people. However, our feeling emotionally unsafe or physically unsafe when we try to discuss our differences may also be an indication of abuse.

Whether you grew up in a confused ignorance of sexuality, an uncomfortable level of exposure, or maybe a confounding mix of both, you deserve to understand your own experiences and process their effects safely. If you know that you were violated sexually as a child or young adult, you may have much stronger emotional and physical responses to this part of the recovery process.

Rather than judge yourself by how calm and collected you wish you were, we encourage you to stay aware of how you are actually feeling and to meet those feelings with care and support. Stress and painful memories can be "reasons" to return to addictive behaviors, so it is important that you take your time, take care, and allow your feelings and memories to move through you slowly, piece by piece, while maintaining the recovery you have already earned.

Identifying and Communicating Boundaries

When someone stands too close to you for comfort, you feel that your physical boundaries have been violated. You may keep stepping back to get the right amount of distance for you. Emotional boundaries operate in the same way. Boundaries say, "This is where you end and I begin."

In families with significant emotional challenges due to addiction, abuse, or other trauma, physical boundaries are often either overly rigid or enmeshed. Rigid boundaries are like walls between caregivers and children. "No one ever touched in my family," one woman told us. "When my parents stood close for photos, it felt so uncomfortable. Remember the invisible shield they used to talk about on toothpaste commercials? That's how it was with my parents and affection—like there was an invisible shield between us." The lack of touch in this woman's family left her feeling distant, isolated, and lonely. As an adult, she felt safe only when she was disengaged and shut down emotionally. She had great difficulty learning how to be intimate.

At the other extreme, families with enmeshed or overly permeable boundaries can lead children into confusion about where they end and others begin. Caregivers with a blurred, unclear sense of their own and others' boundaries can be especially intrusive with their children. This can create an unhealthy form of closeness and intensity of feeling.

One woman told us, "My mother was a psychologist, so you'd think she would have known better. She always wanted to know what I was thinking, what I was feeling. And then she'd analyze my thoughts and explain that I wasn't crabby because I was coming down with a cold, but because I was avoiding my feelings! It felt like she was always inside my head. She imposed her own version of reality onto me, instead of validating and respecting what I was experiencing." Children raised in overly enmeshed families lack a healthy sense of separateness and individuality that might enable them to know and to say what feels okay and what doesn't. They may grow into adults who unconsciously violate others' boundaries and allow others to violate theirs.

Sexual boundaries are often very confusing in families with multiple challenges. Parents may be intrusive and rigid at the same time. Teenagers may lack privacy in the bathroom, yet at the same time be forced to submit to unrealistic regulations about dating. Caregivers may express horror at inadvertent nudity yet tolerate inappropriate touch; some will touch each other and their children with utter impunity.

According to one client, "When I was twelve, my father was always making remarks about my breasts, like that they were bouncing around and I should wear a bra. It was really embarrassing and made me quite self-conscious. But when I tried to talk to my parents about sex, they told me I wasn't old enough to know yet." Confusing messages, confusing silences, and a host of specific rules: It's very difficult for young people to navigate.

Parents may also be intrusive without being rigid, which a child's friends often interpret as being "cool." The parent may think nothing of engaging with their child's social media accounts, becoming friends with their teenager's dates, or drinking with their teenager and their friends. What matters is whether the child feels comfortable with this behavior, or if they are uncomfortable and disempowered, unable to express their boundaries.

Conversely, caregivers can be rigid without being intrusive. They may be disinclined to listen to a young person when they want to talk about what is going on in their life, minimizing their experiences and telling them "Wait until you're older." Rigid but distant caregivers do things like always requiring their daughter to be home from a date at 10 p.m. even if the movie she went to see doesn't get out until 10:15 p.m., and forbidding her to see the person she likes ever again if she is late.

Children who are unclear about sexual boundaries become adults who express confusion about what is appropriate sexual behavior when dating and who may have difficulty saying no to pressure from others. Few parents are able to help their teenagers understand what kind of sexual play is "okay" with a date, because they do not know how to encourage their children to *feel what their own boundaries are*. Even less common are parents who are equipped to help their adolescents develop a sense of appropriate sexual expression when what started as a date progresses into a relationship.

It is important to take a good look at the physical, emotional, and sexual boundaries in your childhood. Where were they? When did you feel they were violated? Did you yearn for more closeness and less rigidity? Or did you need more clearly defined limits? Your answers to such questions may give you insight into how you define your boundaries now and whether you'd like to change them. Boundaries can serve to create both safety and opportunities for intimacy. What might this look like in your own life?

As an adult recovering from an addiction or trauma, you likely are working on identifying and expressing boundaries. Identifying boundaries is the inner work, and expressing those boundaries is the outer work. You may benefit from practicing the following steps:

1. **Notice that you need a boundary and identify what it is.** Boundaries are about limits and protection; we need boundaries to define us and prevent our merging with others in sacrifice of our selfhoods. If your boundaries have been violated repeatedly, you will probably have problems with noticing when you need a boundary. Learning to feel your own boundaries and limits requires tuning in more to your body's sensations, also called mindfulness.

   When do you feel tightness in your chest or throat, a flush of hot or cold, a desire to shake your hands or legs, difficulty getting a full breath, nausea, or the desire to dissociate? Check and see if there is something happening that you want to escape, change, or refuse. In this situation, are you feeling fearful and challenged but are safe to continue? Or are you feeling out of control and unsafe, and you need to take a step back and set a boundary?

   We all have an internal sensor that decides if we are okay or not okay. Sometimes co-author Vanessa calls it a "thumbs up/thumbs down-o-meter." When you begin to feel thumbs-down about a situation, it may be time to set a boundary. The more you are able to listen to your body's sensations, the more information you will have about what is okay with you and what is not okay with you. This ability comes with time and practice. Do not be discouraged if you aren't clear about your body's responses right away.

2. **If appropriate, communicate your boundary to those who may be affected.** This step is challenging especially for survivors of abuse and violence, but once we are living in safer conditions, it is extremely important to practice. Communicating a boundary is different from asking someone else to change their behavior. Boundaries do not control

others; they tell others what we are going to do and what we will not do. "I will not discuss that issue any more today" is a boundary. In contrast, "Stop talking to me about this!" is asking someone else to change their behavior.

There are times when communicating a boundary is not appropriate. You are free to stop communicating with anyone, at any time. Keep in mind that communicating boundaries is part of ongoing relationship, and creating boundaries without communicating them usually means you are stepping back from the relationship.

3. **Offer care to yourself, regardless of others' response to the boundary.** Identifying and communicating boundaries can cause us stress, especially when we first start practicing. We may be overly strident or too meek at first. We may be terrified of what the other person will say or do, especially if we have been violated in the past. No matter what happens, remember that setting boundaries is a skill you can learn, and as you practice, it requires time and self-care afterward. Even if it goes beautifully, take a moment to acknowledge this to yourself. This will help you feel safer the next time.

4. **Take time to consider the boundary, and revise it when appropriate for you.** Sometime after setting a boundary, you may want to go back and consider it more fully. Once you are not in the heat of the moment, maybe you can see why the boundary arose and make clearer choices for yourself about how to proceed. Boundaries are not meant to be cement walls. They are meant to cultivate a feeling of safety for us and the people we are in relationship with. This means they change as we change, and that's a good thing.

Naming the Personal Past

Naming your sexual experiences is crucial to developing honesty about sexuality in recovery. Saying aloud what happened and what didn't happen and naming it appropriately is often a painful process. We must grieve the hurts that have happened to us, and we also must grieve the harm we may have caused others.

As you begin to look at your sexual past, you may find, as Ash did, that you have minimized the abusiveness of your sexual experiences. Ash told their trauma therapist, "I had a lot of sex I didn't want to. I know why I did it, but also, I think I didn't want to feel angry at the people who coerced me into having sex for something I needed from them. I didn't want to believe that they were that selfish, or that I had been abused again and again, long after leaving the home where my stepfather hurt me. It was so depressing to realize that I'd just been in one exploitative situation after another."

It's very important to be able to see something as it really is and to label it according to the words that feel true for you. When Ash was able to name their experience, it helped them see that, yes, they were doing their best to survive a terrible situation for years after the initial childhood sexual abuse, and also that they had been sexually coerced, exploited, raped, and harmed.

Naming the past can be a painful experience. Like many who have been harmed, you may have survived by shutting out the awareness of the reality of your sexual experiences. But as you grow in recovery, you will find that moving beyond old behaviors means telling the truth about where you have been.

If you find that truthfully naming the past brings up unmanageable feelings for you, don't hesitate to seek help. Self-help groups, support groups, and individual therapy can all help to support you in confronting the reality of your past sexual experiences.

Joining a Support Group

Naming your past may be easiest to do while in a recovery group that includes sexuality as an issue. In such a group, many women, nonbinary people, and gender-expansive people feel safe for the first time in their lives to talk about and name what actually happened. You may discover that your experiences with sexuality are similar to others' experiences and that other people in your group know and understand exactly what you are talking about.

"I wasn't sure about joining a women's group," one woman told us. "I thought that because I'm trans, the other women might think I didn't belong. But instead, I felt totally welcomed, and I realized that I wasn't alone in my struggle with alcohol, drugs, and recovering from rape. Sure, cisgender women had different experiences, but they had shame and secrets, and we could connect over those themes. It helped me feel more grounded every time I went."

Being in a group can help remove the tremendous burden of individual responsibility that we often feel about our struggles with sexuality. Many come to see that their addictive behaviors are reactions to abuse, generational traumas, and other issues that are much larger than one person. In a group, we can begin to accept the ways our sexual expression has reflected our self-worth, or our desire to be accepted, loved, and validated.

Unfortunately, many women's and queer recovery groups have an unspoken agreement not to talk about sex. This can send the message that sex must not be important in recovery from substance use issues, since no one's talking about it. Or attendees might fear that no one else is having sexual difficulties and problems, and that there's something very different—broken and wrong—about them.

If you are a member of a group in which sex isn't mentioned, you may need to break the ice by suggesting sexuality as the topic for a particular meeting. This was how Michelle and her group came to discuss sexuality. One of the group members asked if they could talk about childhood sexual abuse after there had been a series of news stories about a celebrity sexual predator. The group rallied around the conversation and opened deeper levels of compassion and recovery.

The peer support group that Nova started often discussed sexual issues because the members were all women, femmes, and nonbinary people who worked in sex-related businesses. Because sex work was a consistent topic of conversation, the group also discussed sexuality outside of work and supported each other through relationship issues, boundary setting, sexual communication, sexual health, and many other topics.

Sexuality is one of the most difficult subjects for people to talk about. But when given the chance, it's amazing what we need to say, want to say, and have to say. If it isn't appropriate for your group, you can seek out another group for additional support that specifically addresses sexuality and relationships.

Some groups are peer led, like Nova's, and some are run by a licensed therapist or other trained facilitator. An online search for "recovery group" plus the issue most important to you can start you in the right direction. You can look for a group that is working through a text, or you can join a recovery meeting for women and see if there is a small group that has formed around sexuality.

Recovery Programs

Because of a new consciousness on the part of many people who are now working in the recovery field, a number of treatment programs are beginning to have regular groups for women and queer people. Depending on the program, these meetings should include trans, nonbinary, and gender-expansive people. Almost invariably, attendees express how important these groups are to their recovery and how appreciative they are of their existence. There is something inherently empowering about a group that focuses on our lives as we experience them.

This empowerment helps us name our experiences truthfully. If you work in a treatment program that has no women's group, you might suggest that one of the regular groups be separated by gender at least once a week. Treatment programs that have created women's groups, and seen how effective they are, have made them a part of their standard program.

Support groups come in all shapes and sizes—some are peer led, some are led by a trained therapist or facilitator. Some are large, and some are small. Some meet in person, others online. Some have a cost, some are free. Some follow a curriculum, and some are just for real-time conversation.

Most recovery programs have directories of meetings and groups, and you can often find offshoots by asking around in those communities. Many therapists have groups they can recommend, and a large number of counselors run groups that have information posted online. You may need to search for a little while to find the right group. Or you can always start one of your own and work through *Awaken Your Sexuality* and the *Awaken Your Sexuality Workbook* together!

◦ ◦ ◦

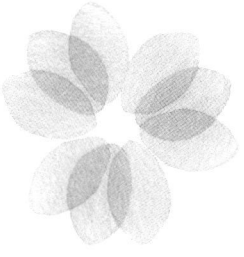

CHAPTER 6

Facing Our Challenges

*When my body feels good, my life feels good,
and I want to keep going, and fight for my
right to exist and love and grow and evolve.
This is true whether it is in the context of
a meeting, or a relationship, or a night of
lovemaking. That doesn't mean the absence
of discomfort or awkwardness or hard
conversations or learning. But the majority
of experience should be presence—being
fully alive. And I think that comes from
experiencing ease, pleasure, connection.
As Nina [Simone] sang: "Feelin' good."*

———

adrienne maree brown, *Pleasure Activism:
The Politics of Feeling Good*

We are rich, complex beings, and for many of us, sexuality is a central facet of this richness. It does not exist in isolation, apart from the rest of life. Our sexuality is affected by everything that affects our mood: stress, anxiety, cravings, sleep, nutrition, social connections, and so on. We can benefit from considering how our sexual feelings may relate to what else is going on in our lives. Recognizing these connections can open up a new level of self-understanding.

When you begin to tell the truth to yourself about your sexual past, to give accurate names to your experiences and relax your judgments of self, you will also begin to look deeper into what you were looking for or seeking to communicate through your sexual behavior. You will begin to acknowledge your longings. Your longings may include to be held, to be touched, to be loved, to be validated, to be in control, to feel excitement, to try something new, to feel safe, to avoid loneliness, to feel connected, to enjoy something, to escape, to feel high, to show love.

As part of the inner journey of recovery, you looked honestly at your sexual feelings and began to deal with your hurt and pain. The outer journey of recovery requires you to look honestly at your adult sexual patterns and to name your experiences.

In this chapter, we will spend some time with a few of the most common challenges we see in the sexual lives of women, nonbinary people, and gender-expansive people who are in recovery from addiction and trauma. These include imbalanced relationship dynamics, sex avoidance, and out-of-control sexual behavior. If you see yourself in these descriptions, you are in great company—the company of people in their own recovery process. Healthy sexuality, as you define it for yourself, begins with honest awareness of your past actions and identification of the values and desires you hold in the present. Then you practice bringing your behavior into alignment with your values and desires.

Power Imbalance in Relationships

Women in our society are socialized to be in imbalanced relationships; that is, we are taught to feel satisfaction and fulfillment from meeting the needs of others, from putting others first in our lives. We come from many generations of women who learned to center their lives around the needs of partners, spouses, children, or aging parents, often at the expense of their own growth, development, and satisfaction. This story is more complex for trans women, nonbinary and gender-expansive people, and women who partner with other women. However, no one is untouched by the dominant gender norms in our society.

Even women who rebel against these norms are affected by them, because they are made to feel like "confrontational" or "selfish" women whose nonconformity is dangerous to everyone. An easy example is the thousands of child-free women sharing their lives on social media, who receive hateful, shaming comments about how they are acting against nature and will never be truly happy. Trans women and many nonbinary people must contend with these expectations of women plus the particular struggles that prejudice against their gender identities brings.

A quick note that for some people, a power imbalance is part of sexual play, as in BDSM. While traditionally seen as an acronym for *bondage, discipline, dominance, submission, sadism, and masochism*, BDSM refers to a wide range of relational and sexual practices that usually involve a clear power exchange among partners. Consensual BDSM can be a great place to practice boundaries, sexual communication, and self-awareness with trusted partners. Power imbalances in relationships *that cause distress* are a very different thing.

In consensual kink, not quite synonymous with BDSM, there may or may not be a power imbalance as part of the experience. *Consensual kink* refers more broadly to sexual practices that fall outside dominant norms. For both kink and BDSM, however, a power dynamic is a conscious choice made by all involved, and among the many feelings it can elicit, satisfaction and pleasure should appear. The power imbalances discussed in this section are very different—they tend to be built over time without discussion, cause significant distress, and create conflict in relationships that makes sexual connection difficult to achieve.

When we do not learn how to define and meet our own emotional needs, we depend on others for our sense of self and self-esteem. We might struggle with setting boundaries because we fear abandonment. Sexually, this may mean consistently putting a partner's sexual needs ahead of our own—engaging in sex without enough arousal, allowing a partner to always decide what type of sex to have, having sex when we're feeling angry, feeling guilty about our own body's response to our partner, and so on.

It is normal to have some trouble identifying and asserting sexual limits and boundaries, because it is normal to have had insufficient or even harmful education about sexuality. Many women who were raised in strict religious households struggle with the concept that they should have any sexual agency at all. Others may simply find it embarrassing to speak up when a partner is doing something that doesn't feel great. In some cases, we learn not to hurt our partner's ego because they may become enraged, punishing, or dangerous.

In a consensual partnership where adults are sharing power, sexual issues are seen as a reason to slow down, get curious, and offer support. Because many of us didn't learn in childhood that we have a right to be treated with dignity and respect, we may have lost the ability to hear, honor, and value our own sexual feelings and desires. We may never have had someone slow down and try to understand our hesitation, fear, or concerns. Pair that history with the socialization of boys and men, which tells them they are entitled to sex when and how they want it, and imbalanced power in the sexual relationship will follow. The issue of power imbalance isn't reserved for heterosexual-type relationships, of course, but it does play out there in a visible and normalized way.

Valuing a relationship does not make you imbalanced; in fact, it creates balance and intimacy. It is a lack of mutuality, the way one partner puts more time and energy into the relationship than the other, that can result in imbalanced relationship dynamics.

In her book *Emotional Labor: The Invisible Work Shaping Our Lives and How to Claim Our Power*, author Rose Hackman describes in deeply researched detail the ways women are expected to provide emotional care and logistical support to the lives of those around them, and what happens when that effort is not acknowledged or adequately reciprocated. Unsurprisingly, the results are that women feel increased stress and resentment.

In other words, if one partner is expected to tend to the needs of the other, and there is not enough reciprocity to keep the relationship balanced, stress and resentment build. It is very difficult to feel turned on, relaxed, honored, and excited about sex if you've been taking care of others all day and don't see an end to it in the bedroom.

Veronica, now in her late seventies, identified herself as a person with a history of imbalanced relationship dynamics. She was raised in the Midwest in a working-class family. Her mother was very passive and had gotten married at eighteen to get away from her own abusive family. Veronica, too, fled from her family through marriage, but also through education. She knew she needed financial stability to get out of what she felt was a stifling environment, so she worked very hard to win scholarships and otherwise earn the means to educate herself. For years she worked as a biologist in a county medical laboratory.

When Veronica looked at her family and how she learned about sexuality, she recognized some familiar patterns:

> I was raised in the 1950s, when nobody, I mean *no-body*, talked about sex. My mother didn't even tell me about menstruation until I came crying to her when I was eleven because I thought I was bleeding to death.
>
> When I got married at nineteen, I was pretty ignorant about my own body and about sex in general. I had masturbated since I was a little girl, and I knew how to have an orgasm, but I didn't know that you could have one with a partner too. During the ten years I was married, I never had an orgasm. I just thought intercourse was different than masturbation. More satisfying in some ways, less in others.
>
> My husband was an alcoholic. I'd drink with him in the evenings. We'd have sex in the missionary position, and I'd fall asleep either high or drunk. The next morning, I'd have a terrific headache, but I always

attributed it to the drinking. It didn't occur to me then that my headache could also have been caused by my frustration and despair and the way I was lying to myself about my life.

I had no idea of learning about and asserting my own sexual desires. I thought that in marriage your job was to please your husband and that you'd better do it, or he'd leave you, and justifiably so. Now I look back at all those headaches I had and say, of course! I must have built up tremendous unreleased sexual and physical tension as well as resentment.

Sometimes we develop addictions or compulsive behaviors to escape the discomfort of our imbalanced relationships. Michelle and Chris, while working through their disconnection in therapy, arrived at a surprising impasse: They both felt that the other person relied on them for too much emotional and physical labor in their family home.

Michelle had identified that her drinking, in addition to other ways it offered her relief, was a way to escape the pressures of motherhood, especially the exhaustion and frustration of being a stay-at-home mom. She felt that Chris expected her to do everything perfectly, like a 1950s housewife, and she was angry with him for not helping more around the house.

To Chris, Michelle had seemed incapable of caring for their home or children the instant he arrived home from work because she was drinking so heavily. He felt responsible for the safety of their children, caring for them when Michelle was drunk at night, when she was out at boozy brunch, or when she was hungover, and then monitoring her for poor decisions when she was with them, even while he was at work. When Michelle quit drinking and began her recovery, she still needed hours away from the children to go to meetings. Even though Chris saw improvement in their home life and was glad Michelle was sober, their relationship still needed deeper communication about their expectations of each other and how they could support each other going forward.

Sex Avoidance

We may feel the need to avoid sex with others for many reasons. Most of them boil down to our sense of safety. If we are not safe to express our sexuality, we will try not to. If our body sends danger signals when someone touches us, we will avoid contact. Sometimes we work on creating more safety for ourselves through sobriety, recovery, therapy, and group support, but we still feel fearful, ambivalent, or avoidant of sexual experiences.

Sex avoidance for a period of time may be called *celibacy* or *abstinence*. There is nothing wrong with taking some time to evaluate your own sexual feelings without engaging in sex with others, like Nova chose for herself. Nova had no plans to remain abstinent from sex for the rest of her life. However, it was a positive experience to take some months to focus on herself and learn more about her body, especially her struggles with methamphetamine addiction and food restriction. She was able to center her own recovery without the pressure of caring for another person's feelings about sex. As Nova experiences changes in her relationships to food and her own body, she may feel more energy available for dating and partnership.

What is important to notice is *how it feels* to release the expectation of sex. If avoiding sex feels good to you, like a weight off your shoulders, then refraining from sexual contact with others may be an experiment in self-awareness and recovery. Like Nova, you may find it a place of freedom and rich, informative experience. You may need the break to reconnect with your own body and feelings before you begin a new sexual relationship or return to a familiar one.

However, if avoiding sex feels distressing to you, then you may want to spend some more time investigating the nature of your avoidance. Some people feel it necessary to avoid sex with others because they have a history of out-of-control sexual behavior. This is much like the need to stop drinking before real recovery can begin to take place. The emotional quality of the avoidance matters. Some people are not fearful; they avoid sex because it simply isn't what they want for themselves. Some wish to be more sexually connected but experience symptoms of trauma when they try: dissociation, freezing, numbing, and so on. If you know you are avoiding sexual contact but aren't sure why, see if any of the following applies to you.

Sexual Orientation

Sometimes sex avoidance is connected to a person's need to discover or express something about their sexual orientation. There is no reason to try to force yourself to be more sexual if you do not experience sexual attraction or the desire to express yourself sexually with a partner. You may be in a totally normal ebb of sexual feeling.

If your whole life has been characterized by this feeling, then you might consider identifying on the asexuality spectrum. It is a myth that asexuality is an illness, a hormone imbalance, or a psychological condition. Asexuality is a sexual orientation, and people who identify as asexual are usually regarded as part of the LGBTQIA+ community.

While some people who identify as asexual avoid partner sex completely, others may still engage in it for various reasons and enjoy it. Because asexuality exists on a spectrum, sex avoidance itself does not mean a person needs to identify as asexual. Identifying as asexual is a personal choice based on how a person feels about their sexuality. If you are interested in learning more about asexuality, a good place to start is Sherronda J. Brown's book *Refusing Compulsory Sexuality: A Black Asexual Lens on Our Sex-Obsessed Culture.*

Awaken Your Sexuality is for women, nonbinary people, and gender-diverse people who are seeking to recover sexually, which means uncovering and experiencing your unique sexuality. For some, this will mean facing that your sexual orientation is not heterosexual: Maybe your addiction or trauma has hidden your asexuality, bisexuality, pansexuality, or lesbian attraction from you.

Recall that this was the case for co-author Stephanie, who had to acknowledge her attraction to women once she stopped drinking. Sexual recovery does not guarantee that your unique sexuality will be socially accepted, personally comfortable, or even totally understandable to you at first. Some people do not experience changes in their sexual orientation over time, while others do. What recovery is about is honest, real-time presence with how you actually feel, and then acting in integrity with your values. For some, this will look like avoiding sex for a time as they consider their true desires.

Social Factors

Social factors often play a role in sexual avoidance. Since so much fear and shame surrounds women's sexuality in general, simply not being sexual may seem to be the easiest course to take. Many women find it extremely difficult to face society's disapproval of women's sexual expression. We are damned if we do, and damned if we don't.

If you are interested in nonnormative sexual practices, including kink and BDSM, you have to navigate a host of subcultural social factors, like the way partner selection in kink is a rather different dance than nonkinky dating. If you are looking to get married to a man and are worried that having sex too soon will ruin your chances with someone, you have to time your "giving in" just right. If you are bisexual and dating a woman, you may feel pressure to continuously prove you are "queer enough." If you have a visible disability, potential partners may fetishize you rather than engage you as a full human being, and you may have to screen potential dates for these dynamics. If you are trans or nonbinary, you may need to create more room for communication about gender in your relationships than you have in the past. The list goes on, and it can be daunting.

For many people, the difficulties of finding partners to be fully present with makes sexual connection feel out of reach. They may begin to suppress their own sexual feeling to avoid more disappointment.

While it may be challenging to meet appropriate partners, get to know them, and get comfortable being sexual without the aid of old substances or habits, it is more than possible. We will revisit this issue in later chapters.

Addiction

Let's start with alcohol. Drinking suppresses the physiological responses of sex organs, which means women who drink to excess may have a harder time being responsive to touch, experiencing physical arousal, and achieving orgasm than nondrinking women. Getting aroused and achieving satisfaction sexually while actively drinking may thus seem futile, and many women just stop trying. Or so much energy may be focused on drinking, controlling drinking, and thinking about the next drink that little energy is left to invest in developing sexual relationships. Some women regularly drink until they pass out, and so are not able to be present for sex.

Sexuality is often one of the first things a woman neglects in order to conserve her time and energy for engaging in addiction behavior. For any addiction, a certain amount of daily life must be reserved for getting the substance or securing the privacy to engage in a behavior.

Different substances affect our sexual response in different ways. Nova spent years using alcohol, cocaine, and methamphetamine to stay awake and party with her clients at the strip club. The cocaine and methamphetamine often made her feel energetic and sexual, but they also suppressed her orgasmic response. She could get excited, but eventually she would feel frustrated, and then she would use alcohol to help her calm down and sleep. This cycle eventually made her feel numb, and it contributed to her confusion about what sexual signals her own body might be sending her.

When we enter recovery, we must face ourselves and our choices. If we have shame about our sexuality or any sexual experience, our sexuality can get bumped to the bottom of the priority list. It is not hard to understand why something that is such a source of conflict is so readily repressed.

Boundary Violation

Boundary violations occur on a continuum, from lack of privacy to covert or emotional abuse and physical abuse. A violation incident need not be sexual to have a negative impact on a woman's sexuality. Sex may feel threatening and unsafe due to one violation or countless violations over time.

Carolyn, a social worker in her mid-thirties, came to therapy because of the lack of sexual expression in her current relationship. She had been sober for six years and had a solid recovery practice in AA, but she was unhappy because she didn't feel very sexual in sobriety and felt there was something missing. She realized that she had always avoided sex, only rarely getting past her avoidance, and then only when drinking.

"My family was a white, middle-class stereotype," she began. "Outside we looked great; we were all talented and successful. We all played sports and were popular at school. But at home, no one seemed to respect the others. After dinner, conflict would become loud, sarcastic, and cruel. I would try to get away, but I never knew when my brothers would barge into my bedroom or the bathroom without knocking. My mother would go through my room, looking for evidence that I was doing drugs or having sex, when I wasn't. I was on eggshells all the time, afraid of getting yelled at.

"When I started having sex, I was scared, and I couldn't even get near someone without a lot of alcohol in me. Even now, after being sober six years, I still have a hard time warming up to someone. I need to be really close to someone to be able to be sexual, so I've only had two partners in my life. I want to feel freer, more relaxed. I feel fear, most of the time."

Carolyn works in a family service agency. About a year ago, she began working with a colleague, Lauren, to develop a grant for a group program. Through the intensity of the research project, they became friends and began to go to dinner and occasional movies together. Carolyn knew Lauren was a lesbian, but their dating lives never seemed to come up. Although Carolyn had had several sexual encounters with women while drinking, she would not allow herself to have any sexual fantasies or feelings about Lauren.

Carolyn said, "I worked with Lauren for nine months before I even considered that I was attracted to her. It felt really scary how much I liked her. Even then, typical of me, I guess, Lauren had to make the first move. She did everything right; she talked to me about how she was feeling and asked if I wanted to go on an actual date. She didn't pressure me into anything sexual and told me I was worth waiting for. I'm so attracted to her now, but I still feel frozen in fear sometimes when she reaches for me. This relationship is important to me. I'd really like to learn how to be more sexual."

Recovering from a lifetime of boundary violations takes time and patience. Carolyn has a great starting point: She has a partner who is invested in going on the journey with her. Learning to be "more sexual" is about learning to be more comfortable with our bodies, our vulnerability, our boundaries, our desires, and our communication.

Out-of-Control Sexual Behavior

Sexual avoidance and out-of-control sexual behavior may seem like opposites, but they are both coping mechanisms for pain in our sexual lives. Women, nonbinary people, and gender-expansive people who have experienced sexual abuse or rape are very likely to choose one extreme or the other as a way to cope with trauma and feel some control over what happens to them. Therapist and author Douglas Braun-Harvey defines *out-of-control sexual behavior* (OCSB) as "a sexual health problem in which consensual sexual urges, thoughts, or behaviors feel out of control."[1]

Note that this does not include sexual assault or rape that happens to a person while they are intoxicated, nor sexual assault or rape that a person may commit while intoxicated. OCSB refers to engaging in sexual behaviors that violate our sexual values, within a framework of consensual experiences. In other words, while our behavior may hurt someone's feelings or cause us distress, the behaviors are not crimes against another person.

Some OCSB occurs as a result of being drunk, high, or dissociated. Once a person begins to recover from their addiction or work through their trauma, their sexual behavior may consequentially change to be more in alignment with their values. Their OCSB was a symptom of the addiction. This was the case for Hannah.

Hannah had experienced a meteoric rise in a major corporation by the time she turned twenty-six. She had been in recovery for a year when she told the following story to her recovery group:

> My most embarrassing example of sexual acting out happened at my company's anniversary conference. It was black-tie, and I started drinking in my hotel room while getting ready. By the time the DJ set started, I'd been drinking steadily for about four hours. I remember dancing, but not much else. The next morning, I was more hungover than usual.
>
> I ran into many co-workers checking out of the hotel and on the shuttle to the airport. The vibe was off. I could feel people looking at me. I found a work friend and cornered her in the airport bathroom.
>
> She had a hard time telling me what I did, but finally I got the picture. I'd tried to make out on the dance floor with another manager while his wife was watching. I told them we should have a threesome, and everyone heard it.
>
> I was mortified. Not only could I not remember what had happened, but everybody else had seen it, and they remembered fine.

Hannah was acutely embarrassed as she recounted her story. The experience had prompted her to seek help for her drinking, and she joined an online group. Her behavior at the party was very different from what she would call her sexual values. Although she was single, she was somewhat introverted and rarely dated.

Once she stopped drinking, Hannah spent most of her time working or going to the gym. After dredging up this story in a meeting, however, she decided it told her something about her sexual feelings. *They might be repressed*, she thought, *but I cannot continue to ignore them, especially when they're in danger of coming out unpredictably and in a form completely disconnected from my values when I'm uninhibited.* She decided to examine this neglected aspect of her life more closely.

Another type of OCSB continues to persist even in sobriety from alcohol and other substances. This is what people often call "sex addiction." There are many recovery communities who find it the best description of their experience, and many people feel seen and supported by identifying with the term. Rather than engage in the debate about the validity of this term, we would like to honor those who use it to describe their own feelings and behaviors, while using the term *OCSB* to encompass all those who have had sexual behavior that felt out of control. For example, some people find that once they are sober from drugs, alcohol, or other behaviors, sex becomes the arena where they act out impulsively or compulsively, maybe for the first time. They may not identify as "sex addicts," but they are concerned about their behavior nonetheless.

There is no specific definition for what an "out of control" behavior is—for one person, having more than twenty partners in a year may feel out of control, while for another, that feels perfectly normal. For one person, engaging in consensual kink with a professional dominatrix may feel safe, while for another, it feels out of control. For nonmonogamous people in consent-based relationships, having multiple partners at once may feel normal. For a monogamous person who is cheating, having multiple part-ners at once is likely going to feel out of control. Aside from the basics of mutual consent, you are the only one who knows what your values are and when you are in violation of them. Consider the following questions:

- What do I want when I want sex?
- What kind of sexual partner(s) do I want to have?
- How comfortable am I speaking openly about sex with my partner(s)?
- What level of sexual risk am I comfortable with?
- Would my former partners say I was interested in their boundaries and got appropriate consent from them for our sexual experiences?
- Would I say my former partners have been interested in my boundaries and got consent from me for our sexual experiences?

OCSB is not the same thing as the experience of an out-of-control relationship, but they can occur at the same time. Again, for many people the word *addiction* feels most appropriate for the experience, while for others, *compulsive*, *impulsive*, or *out of control* feels truer.

We had an illuminating conversation with best-selling author Elizabeth Gilbert, who identifies as a recovering sex and love addict and who is also sober from all mind- and mood-altering substances. Years of therapy and other approaches were somewhat helpful to Elizabeth; however, she now participates in a Twelve Step program that has finally offered her the kind of support she needed most. For Elizabeth, the term *addiction* has many layers of meaning.

She told us, "My relationships have always begun in tremendous passion and ended in tremendous shame. They've almost always overlapped. And anybody who was looking at my romantic and sexual resumé and life history would say, this is a person who is not well. I knew it. I went to therapy for years about it, but nobody ever used the word *addiction*. Interestingly, in the pages of *Eat, Pray, Love*, I used the word *addiction*. That was twenty years ago! I used the language of addiction to describe what happens to me in infatuation and obsession, but I still didn't know that there was such a thing as a sex and love addict. I think I'd heard of sex addiction, but I associated it with men, with a particular kind of behavior that didn't look like what my behavior looked like."

For Elizabeth, "sex and love addiction" is a framework that helped her change her life through a spiritual solution. She is currently abstinent from sexual and romantic relationships, and she has found great freedom and peace in the process. Elizabeth told us, "I have a life that has a lot of pleasure in it now. And I didn't before. I had a life that had a lot of sex in it. I had a life that had a lot of orgasms in it. It was like a buffet! But like a buffet on a cruise ship.

"Ultimately, that is not the same thing as pleasure. The neediness that I never stopped experiencing is the exact opposite of pleasure. For me, pleasure cannot exist without serenity. Serenity, for me, cannot exist in the state of need. So pleasure and need are two very different things. Even saying to somebody 'I need pleasure; I need you to pleasure me' means I'm already very far from pleasure. The amount of cortisol and adrenaline that is running through my veins when I'm demanding or needing that, or trying to get it, is actually not enjoyable."

Elizabeth's experience is both particular to her and holds insights for many. The constant intrigue of looking for and seducing a new person can temporarily reduce anxiety and stress as well as increase your feelings of power and confidence. Women often report using seduction as a way to feel good about themselves.

This was true for Elizabeth, and also for Nova, who decided to take a break from dating and sexual relationships after a few years of sobriety from alcohol and amphetamines.

Without constant validation from men, Nova sought to find love and support in other places. She told her friends that on a good day, she felt beloved and held by them, and able to offer herself care and support, and on a bad day, she turned to her social media for validation. While addressing her eating disorder, she sought to reduce her dependence on others for her self-worth.

Ultimately, this is the task for everyone in recovery: to determine the best way to act in alignment with your values. As Elizabeth told us, "Before recovery, I wouldn't say I knew peace. Now, I know it is rare, but I also know what it feels like and how to cultivate it."

The Sexual History Lifeline

Filling out a Sexual History Lifeline is an effective way to see how your sexual behavior has been shaped by your life experiences, including your addictions or compulsive behaviors. Figure 2 is an example, reflecting Ash's experiences. Figure 3 is an empty chart for you to fill out, or you can use the Sexual History Lifeline in the *Awaken Your Sexuality Workbook*.

The Sexual History Lifeline starts with the bottom horizontal line: from zero to the age you are now, in five-year increments or whatever increments you'd prefer to use. Along the side, there is a vertical line that starts at -10, counts up to 0, and then continues up to 10. This is the measure of whether an experience was positive or negative for you. As you draw your sexual history over the years into this chart, you can label any experiences that are especially meaningful.

After you have charted your sexual history, you can add another line (dotted or in another color) that charts your history with problematic substance use, disordered eating, other self-harming behavior, or significant trauma symptoms.

In the case of substances or addictive behaviors, it may be challenging to decide how "positive" or "negative" an experience was, given the confusing way our substances and addictive behaviors make us feel better in the short term. Use your best judgment in the present. In general, you may assume that times of out-of-control use would be shown as dipping low on the chart.

When you look back through your past to identify your sexual experiences, you may remember incidents that you had forgotten, or you may be surprised at how poignant many of your memories are. You may also become aware of certain patterns, especially in the way your sexual history and your history with addiction or compulsive behaviors interact. Seeing how the lines intertwine, the ways they affect and reflect each other, can provide insight into how your sexual behavior and substance use or other out-of-control behaviors have accompanied you in your life. Understanding this connection greatly enhances your ability to create the kind of sexual life you want in recovery.

Explanation of Ash's Sexual History Lifeline

Figure 2 shows Ash's Sexual History Lifeline. Ash has drawn a line with the years of their life marked off at five-year intervals. The space above the line has been designated for pleasant experiences (marked from 1 to 10), and the space below has been designated for painful ones (marked from -1 to -10). Ash has indicated their sexual experiences with a solid line and their alcohol/drug experiences with a dotted line.

Ash begins by charting their sexual history with a solid line. Ash remembers masturbating at age three. It is a positive, pleasurable experience, guilt-free because they didn't yet have a name for what they were doing.

By age four, Ash was experiencing sexual abuse from their stepfather, which included a violent rape at age ten. During this time, Ash dissociated from their body to self-protect.

From ages ten to fifteen, Ash engaged in constant experimental sexual behavior. Some was enjoyable, but some was scary or uncomfortable. Around this time, their self-esteem began to be connected to being attractive to boys, even though they didn't feel like a feminine girl.

Between the ages of fifteen and eighteen, Ash had a variety of sexual experiences, often with older boys or men in some position of power, like the staff member at their group home. Once they were out of the group home, Ash continued to have sex to get basic needs met. They are not sure how many partners they had during this time. They lived with a group of other queer youth who were sharing a motel room, using drugs, and trading sex to get by.

At twenty-three, Ash spent three months in jail, got sober in a rehabilitation stay, and came out as nonbinary. They briefly entered a relationship with a woman. This was a mostly positive experience for Ash, even though they prefer to date and have sex with men.

For the next four years, Ash moved in and out of recovery and return to use. They worked many different jobs and dated new people but struggled to enjoy being sexual while sober. At twenty-six, Ash experienced sexual violence that triggered a difficult depression.

At twenty-seven, Ash met Ben. The relationship was fun, respectful, supportive, and sexy for a year before Ash began experiencing panic attacks and nightmares.

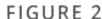

FIGURE 2

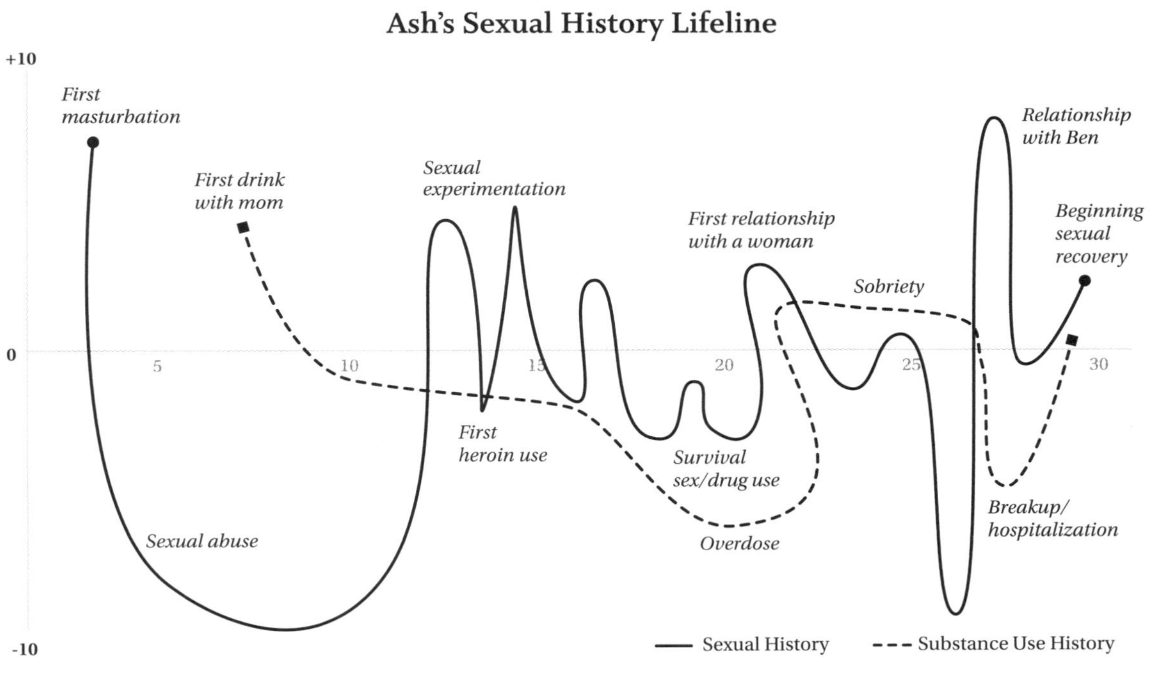

Ash's Sexual History Lifeline

First masturbation

Sexual abuse

First drink with mom

Sexual experimentation

First heroin use

First relationship with a woman

Survival sex/drug use

Overdose

Sobriety

Breakup/ hospitalization

Relationship with Ben

Beginning sexual recovery

+10

0

-10

5

10

15

20

25

30

—— Sexual History

--- Substance Use History

During a psychiatric emergency, Ash was hospitalized and then released without a coherent treatment plan. Ash returned to using familiar substances. Ben broke off the relationship. Ash has not had a sexual partner since that breakup. However, their sexual recovery has progressed. Ash is now able to masturbate without triggering a fear response in their body, so their line is turning upward.

Next, Ash charts their relationship to substance use with a dotted line. They remember their first sip of beer and drag off a cigarette at age six. This is one of the few memories they have with their mother, who died before they were out of foster care.

Ash recalls drinking their mother and stepfather's alcohol in secret at age eight, and then trying to get older men to buy them alcohol after school once they were in foster care.

Ash's first experience with heroin happened at age sixteen, with a boy from school who had stolen it from his sibling. Ash knew it was the drug their mother used and was curious to see why she would choose the drug over her own children. What began as casual use became more serious over the years.

By eighteen, Ash was using heroin and alcohol daily. Their use had ebbs and flows, depending on their financial situation or their health. They had a terrifying experience of overdose at twenty-one, but a friend used naloxone to revive them, and Ash tapered down their use for about a year.

When they were arrested for driving under the influence and without a license, Ash wasn't at the peak of their heroin use, and they were getting tired of the way their life was going. During their three months in jail, they received support from other sober women. They sought treatment. During that transformational time, Ash became ready to say publicly that they were a nonbinary person. They wanted to use they/them pronouns and be referred to by the name *Ash* instead of their legal name. Ash had trouble plotting this period on the chart as either positive or negative, because while it was terrible to be locked up and scary to seek treatment, it was also an important time for their sobriety and self-identity.

At twenty-four, Ash had been in recovery for a year and was stuck on the Fourth Step because they hadn't spoken with their sponsor about their history of sexual abuse. They dropped out of Alcoholics Anonymous and had some fluctuation in their use. During a period of sobriety at twenty-seven, they met Ben.

After their psychiatric emergency and hospitalization, Ash returned to use. When Ben broke up with them, Ash became homeless again. Finally, they returned to recovery with a renewed sense of dedication, and after three years of sobriety, they became a peer counselor.

Ash started working with a trauma therapist to specifically address their history of sexual abuse, unwanted sex, and out-of-control sexual behavior. They have not yet begun a new sexual relationship with anyone, but they are starting to feel more capable of communicating about their sexual feelings and desires.

EXERCISE

Your Sexual History Lifeline

Now you can fill in the blank chart according to your own experiences. The patterns that emerge on the chart can provide the information you need to begin to change those patterns today as a part of your recovery.

FIGURE 3

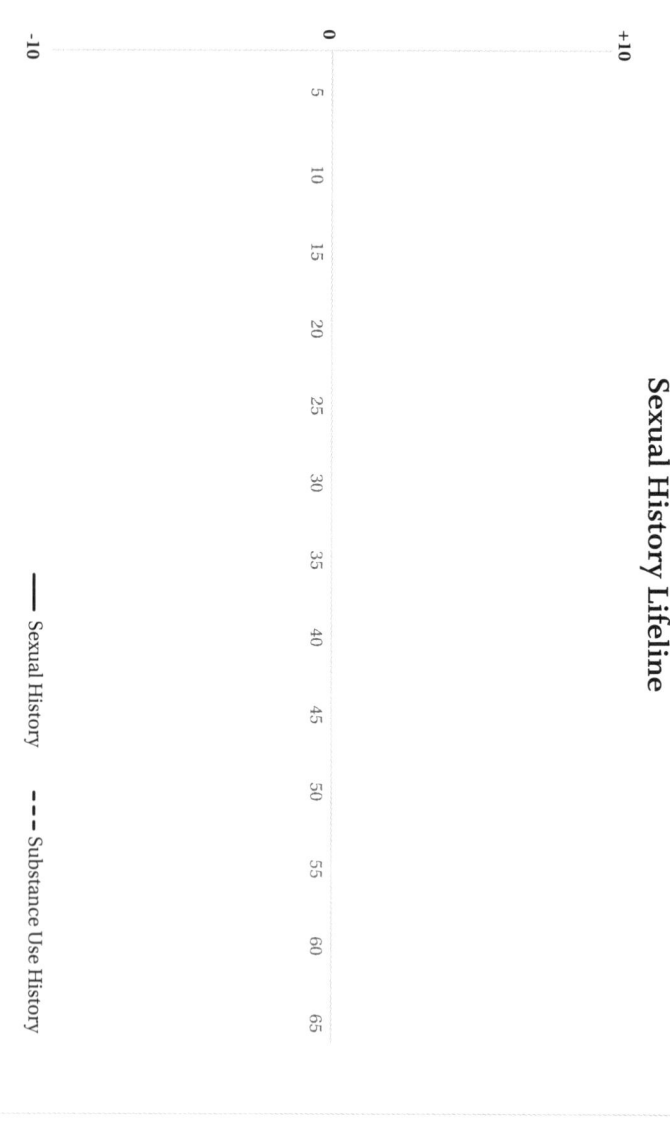

Sexual History Lifeline

——— Sexual History   - - - Substance Use History

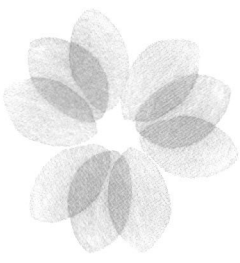

CHAPTER 7

How We Chose Our Partners

SHOULD YOU SEND THAT TEXT

Don't ask me. I'm terrible at it.
Last week I posed the same
question to a friend, who said

"There is nothing in it for you."
But I am in it. "Okay," she said.
"Set an alarm for two weeks

and then see how you feel."
Great advice, I said. I waited
two hours. All my alarms

were going off. So I sent it
and felt victorious and hid
under the bed next to

a dog toy, some dust and
what do you think? Is it love?

———

Jillian Weise (aka Cy), *Cyborg Detective*

.

Whether we do it consciously or unconsciously, by actively seeking or passively accepting, we do choose our sexual relationship partners. Looking at the behaviors of people we have chosen over the course of our lives can be very revealing.

Many of us have told ourselves stories about our partners that minimize their harmful behavior, in the same way we might try to minimize our own. For example, a partner who constantly criticizes you is not seen as emotionally abusive, but is correcting you for your own good. A husband who spends almost every night "out with the boys" is not leaving you in isolation; he is just blowing off steam. The lover who demands you spend every moment together is not trying to control your time or other relationships, she's just madly in love with you. The boyfriend who showed up at your work to make sure you weren't flirting with anyone has been hurt many times in the past, so it's understandable. It can be painful to investigate the past and see all the justifications we made for behavior that was uncomfortable for us.

At other times, we may have been seeking healthy, safe partners with whom we could find refuge. This was how Ash came to view their relationship with Ben. After years of dating people who were not caring for Ash's feelings or well-being, Ash had done enough recovery to start seeking a partnership based on mutual respect, humor, and care. Ben genuinely loved Ash, and so when Ash began experiencing severe mental health symptoms, Ben did his best to be there for Ash.

It wasn't until Ash became violent and returned to using alcohol and heroin that Ben hit his limit and had to leave the relationship. Grieving the loss of Ben and their relationship was part of Ash's recovery process, as was recognizing all the positive traits the relationship had. Ash told a sober friend, "I got really close to what I want with Ben. I will probably miss him for a long time. I'm trying to see it as a sign that I can get even closer to the kind of love I want with another person when I'm ready."

It is as important to take a long, careful look at your partners' behavior as it is to look at your own behavior. This is not because you can change them or control what they do, but because you can see where you need to adjust your own boundaries and communication.

You may feel more inclined to look at your own behavior because you have control over changing it. You may wonder what good it could possibly do you to name the behavior of people with whom you've been intimate, especially in the past. But at least two good things can come out of it. First, even though you have no control over your partners' behavior, now or in the past, you can better identify how their behavior affected you; and second, you can work on increasing your experience of safety and connection via communicating your boundaries, values, and feelings now and going forward.

If you are currently in a relationship, you may fear that looking honestly at your partner would require you to change the relationship. Before you choose to avoid looking honestly at your current partner, though, realize that honesty doesn't mean you have to make immediate changes. It simply requires you to tell the truth about what's happening now. Telling the truth allows you to assess your options, to see that there are choices. Then you can make the decisions that will help you to take care of yourself.

If you are not in a relationship right now but are actively dating or would like to be in a relationship in the future, this chapter can help you identify those patterns you do not wish to repeat, consider what behaviors you need to be aware of, and identify what feels good to you in a partnership.

If you are nonmonogamous, partner selection may require even more consideration, as your relationships will all be mutually affected by the health and quality of each.

If you are not in and do not plan to be in a relationship, taking a look at your past can still inform you about your beliefs and habits.

Regardless of your relationship status, looking at how you have chosen to be in relationship will help you make clearer, more grounded choices going forward.

Many people in the addiction recovery field believe that early recovery is not a good time to make major relationship changes. The logic is that you need time to focus on and adjust to your recovery, to find out what your needs are. If you are already partnered, you need time to see how your partner responds to the changes you are making. If you aren't, you need time to attain some stability and equilibrium on your own. There is wisdom in this for people who are in relationships that are not abusive. Again, seeing what is true about your partner right now, or re-membering partners in the past, is not the same thing as taking action to end or change a relationship. You can take your time.

There is an exception to this guideline for relationships that are abusive. Staying in an emotionally, physically, or sexually abusive dynamic without supportive interventions will inevitably lead to more harm. Perhaps your partner is causing harm to you most often. Perhaps you are causing harm to your partner because of behavior patterns you have not yet been able to change, or maybe you and your partner both exhibit harmful behaviors toward each other. If you know you are in an abusive relationship but are not yet ready to leave, your focus should be on creating as much safety in the relationship as you can, right now, and making plans for an exit whenever you are ready.

You likely have ideas for how to slow down the harm, like taking breaks during arguments. At the same time, you may need to be researching resources, saving up money for moving costs, or talking to a trusted friend or family member who can help you leave when you are ready.

Women are at the most risk of violence right after leaving an abusive relationship, so a clear safety plan with support outside the relationship is necessary. If you are unsure of what you need in your safety plan, you can call the hotlines listed at the end of this chapter or check the Resources section at the back of the book for some suggestions.

Whatever the qualities and behavior patterns of your relationships, seeing the choices you made with your partner with clarity can only aid in helping you become a healthier sexual person.

The Ideal Lover vs. Reality

While swiping on dating apps, introducing ourselves in meetings, or scanning whatever room we are in, we often look for those who seem to fit our image of the ideal lover. Many dating coaches will encourage single people to make a list of traits they are looking for in a partner, as well as a list of deal-breakers. We carry our lists inside us and measure new people up. Some of us can fall in love at first sight. (They are perfect! They check all the boxes!)

And often we fall out of love just as precipitously. (They weren't perfect. That means it wasn't meant to be.)

As we come to know the people we date better and better, they become real individuals to us, so that we can no longer project our ideal onto them. Eventually, we either move on or choose to build a more conscious relationship.

If you feel your partner is ideal, perfect, and therefore better than you, it's time to sit down and consider that your perception of them may be out of sync with who they are. If you feel your partner is not measuring up to your ideal, it is worth thinking about whether the ideal is attainable. New relationships can rely on chemistry, vibes, and novelty. Relationships that last longer require a more intentional investigation of shared values, consistent and honest communication, and mutual support for growing and changing.

Remember that all people are contradictory and complex, including you! We recommend that you keep your eye out specifically for the following patterns you may see in the partners you have chosen.

Partners Struggling with Addiction

When we are actively involved in our substance addiction, compulsive behavior, or trauma symptoms, we may look for companions to be addictive with, not intimate partners who are in their own process of growth and recovery. When you put in the work to change your addictive patterns and get into recovery, you may find some prior relationships floundering because the addiction, not the person, has been the basis for choosing the relationship.

Those of us who grew up in families with big challenges, like parents with addictions, childhood sexual abuse, or other trauma, can often see dysfunctional ways of relating to others as being normal. We carry the burden of generational pain and destructive coping mechanisms, and we often choose partners who have similar struggles.

Current research estimates that children of alcoholics are about four times more likely to develop alcohol problems and are at higher risk of many other behavioral and emotional struggles. This does not mean you cannot change the course of your own life; indeed, it is only you who can do it. Knowing your history is part of developing the self-compassion you'll need to make real change. Your partner deserves to know their own history too.

Maintaining your recovery while staying with an actively using partner is difficult, if not impossible. People struggling with their own addictions or compulsive behaviors are not likely to maintain emotional or sexual availability in relationships. You may begin to feel there is no room in their life for you and your needs. You are not the priority; yours is not the primary relationship in that person's life.

Navigating this impasse can feel excruciating. Telling yourself the truth about how you feel is the most important first step. Are your partner's behaviors making it more difficult for you to recover? Are they willing to begin taking an honest look at their own habits? What would you need to see from them to feel hopeful about this relationship?

Take heed of your answers here, because many of us will slow down or even sabotage our own recovery in the process of trying to support our partner's. This self-sacrifice can also prevent partners from being truly present in relationships. When one partner is constantly focused on anticipating and meeting the needs of the other, there can be no real give-and-take, no emotional growth that comes from authentic mutuality. You cannot single-handedly save another person from their addiction or trauma. They cannot save you from yours.

Unavailable or Emotionally Distant Partners

People can be distant and emotionally unavailable in many ways. For example, they may be cheating on someone. If they are ethically nonmonogamous, they may be managing more relationships than they have capacity for. They may have rigid boundaries that preclude intimacy. They may be depressed and unable to show up for you. They may be self-absorbed and unable to connect with your experience because they are always too distracted by their own.

Distant and unavailable partners may have good reasons for the way they behave, but those reasons are their responsibility to address. Your responsibility is to recognize that you are not experiencing the depth of connection you desire in a relationship, and to make decisions about how you want to proceed. An emotionally unavailable partner will not and cannot bring equal sharing, intimacy, and commitment to the relationship until they are more emotionally grounded and available to do so.

Sometimes partnership with an emotionally unavailable person can feel like an acceptable arrangement, if the expectations can be adjusted to fit the reality. We all have seasons of unavailability due to the events in our own lives.

Adults often live parallel lives at the same address, without attempting to be vulnerable or emotionally present for each other, and this can end up feeling safe for them. However, relationships based in intimacy and mutual understanding cannot sustain that level of distance for long. Only you know if it has been too long for you.

As her recovery progressed, Tamara began to understand that she had become the emotionally unavailable partner to her ex-wife, Alisha. Originally, Tamara felt blindsided by Alisha's request for divorce. She was hurt and angry and felt that Alisha had not tried hard enough to stay together. After a year of recovery from her addiction to painkillers, while using alternative forms of pain management and processing her emotions with a therapist, Tamara developed new insights.

She said, "When Alisha told me she wanted a divorce, I was stunned and went into a deep depression. I thought we had it all worked out. I knew we weren't madly and passionately in love anymore, but we had worked out a life, and I was proud of us being the only middle-aged Black lesbian couple in our small town! I worked long hours at the university, she had plenty of friends to spend time with after she came home from work, and she believed in my mission and purpose, so she never complained about how often I wasn't home. She worried about my health, but she never told me she was unhappy.

"Now I see that we simply lived our own lives and left each other alone. We never talked about anything more serious than what to have for dinner or who was bothering us at work. She definitely tried—I remember nights when she would open up conversations about having sex or having more romance, and I would shut her down. I was too caught up in my work and dealing with my pain from the accident. I thought she would wait for me to get better. I thought we had time to fix whatever she thought was a problem. I didn't realize that I was withdrawing from her emotionally and sexually for years." Tamara withdrew from connection with Alisha, and while Alisha tried to pursue Tamara for a time, eventually it was too hurtful for her, and she decided she needed to end their marriage.

Alisha's initial response to Tamara's withdrawal, which was to ask for more connection, is understandable. A common response to a distant partner is to become a pursuer. As our partners move away, fearing closeness, we rush after them, fearing abandonment and loss. This can happen over and over again, creating a robust pattern. That pattern can last a long time. Eventually, Alisha was the one to break it.

In one of Tamara's women-only meetings, a friend named Rebecca shared that she was often the person chasing a potential partner:

> For years, I thought the problem was men. My girlfriends and I would complain endlessly about them and how they were so afraid of commitment. You'd have a great date, they'd promise to call, and you'd never hear from them again.
>
> When I got into therapy, I began to see that I might actually have a part in the problem. The minute I met a man online, I started fantasizing that he was The One. Then I'd think there could never be anyone better than him, how lucky I was to have found him, and how we would get married and have a wonderful life. Then I'd rush on to the depressing idea that he could leave me, that maybe he really didn't like me at all, that he had another girlfriend he wasn't telling me about. All this in the space of about an hour, waiting for him to text back!
>
> By the time we met in person, I'd be frantic. I'd have run through the entire relationship in my head all the way to its horrible end before it had even started. Because I "knew" he would leave me, I guess I clung hard while he was there. No wonder guys kept running away!

Through sharing her struggle with a support group, Rebecca eventually learned to stop moving forward so fast in order to allow her partners the space to move forward themselves. She needed to slow down and bring herself back to the present, to look at what was happening moment to moment with clear eyes rather than imposing a dark fantasy on events yet to come. When she was able to slow down, she could enjoy getting to know her dates much more. She worked on asking for what she wanted more clearly, and sharing her feelings more honestly with the people she was getting to know.

An important question to reflect on is whether you are more likely to fear abandonment or to fear engulfment. If you have found yourself in this exaggerated dance of pursuer and distancer, you likely have a tendency toward one of these roles. Do you feel terrified when you imagine someone doesn't care for you the way you care for them? Or do you feel afraid that someone will fall for you, expect too much, and you'll have to get away from them?

One reassuring part of this pattern is that as the pursuer learns to pull back, the distancer often moves forward to fill the space. Distancers can reassure their partners that they don't intend to abandon them. Pursuers can benefit from slowing down their future-fantasy thinking and taking stock of what is true in the relationship, right now. Open communication about what each partner is experiencing is key.

Partners Who Abuse

There are many ways to describe and define abuse. Rather than list the behaviors of others that "qualify" as abuse, we encourage you to look inward to define for yourself what behaviors have made you feel demeaned, diminished, disrespected, and harmed. Physical abuse crosses a clear line. What about emotional abuse? Financial abuse? Cyber or online abuse? Stalking?

It may be difficult to understand from the outside, but we do tend to repeat familiar childhood patterns, even if they were humiliating and painful. They are an integral part of who we are and how we learned to behave and understand the world. Some people who experienced childhood abuse even come to feel that they are so bad that they deserve abuse and are not worthy of respect. This is never true.

Self-help groups, groups that focus on recovery from abuse, and individual therapy can be of great help to people who come from abusive backgrounds. The truth is that anyone can find themselves in an abusive relationship. Most of the time it develops slowly. Recognizing the patterns that seem to repeat in your relationships is a major task of sexual recovery, especially if you recognize that there has been abuse.

Partners who abuse fall into roughly two categories: those who recognize that they are abusing and take action to get help to change their behaviors, and those who do not. If your partner is not willing to seek help and make changes, or *says they will but never follows through*, there's a good chance the relationship will remain in an abusive cycle. Not all partners who abuse will escalate from verbal to physical or sexual violence, but many do.

Someone who is being abused will usually do whatever they can to cope and survive. Sometimes a person being abused finds ways to stop a particular situation from escalating further, and so they feel hopeful that the abuse could stop. They may carefully tend to the needs and desires of the abusive partner, apologize for actions that may not have been their fault to appease the abusive partner, or reassure the abusive partner that everything is fine so they will stay in a "good" mood.

When these types of actions seem to work temporarily, they reinforce a belief that we can control the level of abuse a partner will perpetrate, which we ultimately cannot. Some abusive relationships are quite stable, lasting for years. Some abusive relationships are intermittently volatile, including breakups, time apart, and reconciliation.

It is common for partners who abuse to enter a state of vulnerability and instability after they have hurt someone. A person who is being abused begins to walk on eggshells, feels afraid of another crisis, and starts spending their energy trying to make sure their partner is happy. The abusive partner may issue apologies, promise to change, or minimize what happened so all can go "back to normal." When the next crisis comes, the partner who is being abused tries even harder to fix it and return to homeostasis. The longer the relationship, the more the abusive partner needs to ensure loyalty and secrecy, to avoid accountability or the risk of being abandoned by the person they are hurting.

People who have never been inside abusive relationship dynamics do not understand how impossible it feels to end or change them. The longer it goes on, the more difficult it is to leave, for both emotional and practical reasons. Many abusive partners manipulate finances or family relationships to cut off means of escape. Gaining control over another person can be a long game, and partners who are being abused often tell themselves they are fine with making changes for their partner as they slowly relinquish their autonomy. The high of the reconciliation after an explosion can feel incredible, like you have vanquished a demon together and are deeply in love.

Recognizing the reality of abuse can feel embarrassing, shameful, and isolating because of how much stigma victims must endure. In addition, many abused partners eventually take action in retaliation and end up behaving in abusive ways themselves, once they have been backed into a corner. When an abusive partner can say "You're no better than I am" and we believe it, the relationship is even harder to leave.

Co-author Vanessa experienced multiple abusive relationships over many years. They kept the abuse as secret as possible from family and friends, hid their injuries, increased their drug use, and became more prone to reactive behaviors. Finally, after a series of increasingly dangerous instances of physical and sexual abuse, they were able to make a decision toward recovery.

A few years later, they were sharing some of their experience with family at a holiday gathering. A family member wanted to know why it was that Vanessa had been choosing abusive partners. In essence, the question was "What's wrong with you that you let people treat you this way?"

Stigmatizing questions aimed at survivors of violence do not help survivors reflect on our experience. If anything, they make us feel defensive, unheard, and alone. In addition, questions aimed at survivors are usually focused on the wrong issue. It is no secret why many of us get caught up in the web of abusive relationships—they are common, they are socially normalized, and we are not supported culturally in our healing from them.

Most abusive relationships start with small, excusable behaviors. They start with a partner who has a strong opinion and does a little bullying. That behavior is often seen by others as smart, powerful, dominant. The real question is not "What's wrong with people who get abused?" but "What's wrong with our society, that we let abusive behavior run rampant and do not interrupt cycles of violence?"

The answers are right in front of us, but because they are societal issues, they are complex and difficult to solve. What we can do here and now is break the cycles we are in and refuse to remain in relationships that harm us. We can also begin to see the signs of disrespect, control, and instability in our partnerships earlier and make clearer boundaries about the behaviors we will and will not tolerate.

This is why it is so important to develop the capacity to feel your own feelings, to sense when you are afraid, disrespected, dismissed, or hurt. Some treatment programs have special aftercare groups for women who are struggling with abusive relationships.

There are many choices to make once you have decided to prioritize your safety. We recommend using the hotlines listed at the end of this chapter and getting in touch with an advocacy group. They provide practical advice for how to deal with the police and the legal system, should you choose to pursue a restraining order or other legal options. They will also help you plan how to get support from your family, your friends, your place of worship, or other community resources. Most of all, they can assist you in creating alternatives for yourself, such as finding places and people to sustain you during the process of extricating yourself from an abusive partner.

Your Relationship Patterns

When you begin to identify trends and patterns in your sexual relationship history and in your family tree, you will learn what you need to do in a program of sexual recovery. A relationship chart and a family map can be used to identify your relationship patterns. They are tools that can help you identify your relationship history and empower you to make new choices.

EXERCISE

The Family Map

The family map is a diagram of the relationships that exist between you and your family members. You decide who belongs on the map—if you were raised by multiple people, in foster care, or in another nontraditional family structure, choose the people with whom you had the most contact.

The family map is a visual tool that represents the relationship patterns you were born into, and it can help you get information on your emotional history. Arati's family map is an example to aid you in drawing and analyzing your own. You may also complete a version of this activity in the *Awaken Your Sexuality Workbook*.

Instructions for the Family Map

The center circle represents you, and the larger circle is where you will draw your map. Draw circles that represent each member of your family, or the people who were significant in your childhood. Use the key to draw lines between you and your family members that describe your current relationship with each person. If you'd like, you can also draw lines between the other circles to represent the relationships your family members have with each other.

Arati's Family Map

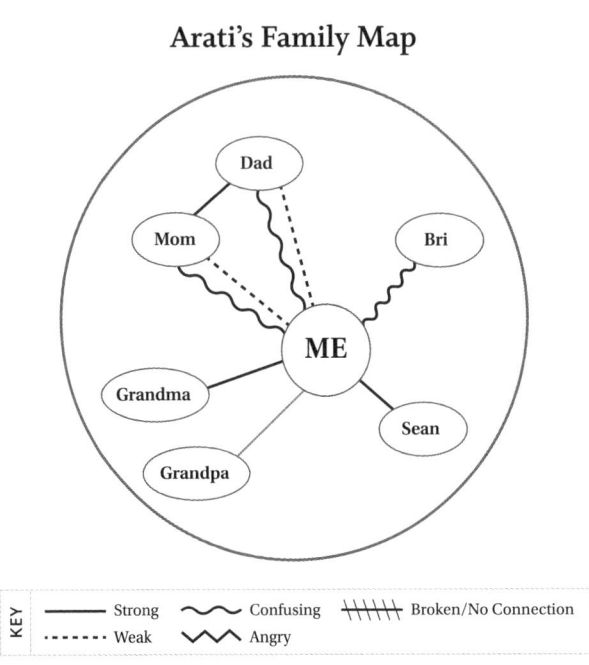

Explanation of Arati's Family Map

Arati drew her immediate family, including her mom; her dad; her sister, Bri; and her son, Sean. Although she had aunts and uncles who were close, she chose to keep her map simple at first. She used dotted and wavy lines to show that her relationships with her parents felt weak and confusing—weaker with her father, more confusing with her mother. Then she added a wavy line to connect to her sister as well. She drew a strong line of connection to her son. She added her grandparents to the map and drew a strong line of connection to her grandmother, with a slightly lighter line to her grandfather.

Looking at her map, Arati realized that, before she had her son, she would have drawn a strong line of connection to her mother and father. She felt sad to recognize this change. When Arati imagined adding a new partner to this map, she envisioned someone who would be able to connect with both her son and her parents.

Arati also recognized that her relationship with her sister was not as close as it might be. They tended to rely on their parents for reasons to see each other, and both lived very busy lives. Bri did reach out regularly to check in on Arati's son, Sean, and Arati felt that trying to share more of her life with her sister could feel supportive. She wondered how her sister's map would look.

Arati perceived her parents' relationship to be very strong, so she drew a strong line of connection between them. However, she realized that she didn't really know what their connection was like with her sister, or with her grandparents. Her family was consistent in fulfilling obligations, marking holidays, and gathering together on special occasions, but that didn't give her the information she was looking for now. She also knew that their extended family would provide a lot more complexity to the map.

What Arati took from this exercise was that deep emotional connection was not taught to her in her family as much as the values of fulfilling familial duty. As a queer woman, Arati knew that she was going to have to create her own path to fulfilling relationships that didn't look like her parents' or grandparents'.

She was grateful for the consistent presence of her family, but she longed for stronger connections that she could rely on emotionally. She wanted to be her full self: mother, inquisitive mind, bisexual partner, recovering woman. Her strong feelings of confusion and nervousness about dating someone new made more sense to her, and she was able to feel some compassion for herself. By putting energy into her own recovery and expressing her sexuality, she was doing something she had not seen before in her own family.

Your Family Map

Now, you can draw a family map using your own experiences.

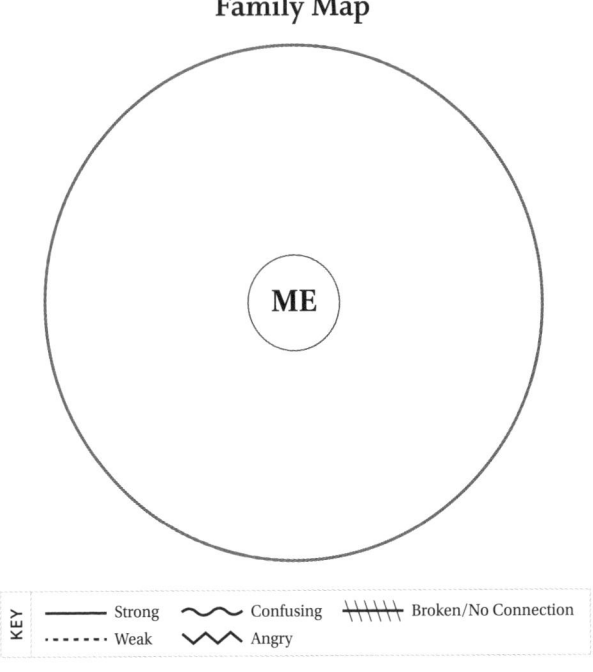

The Relationship History Chart

The Relationship History Chart will give you a picture of who you are in a sexual relationship. This should illuminate how you have developed as a partner, and which patterns and traits you might be repeating. By studying the chart, you can get clues of what you need to do for sexual recovery. You will see the way you interact in relationships and the kinds of partners that you choose. Certain themes, feelings, and characteristics are bound to emerge as patterns. As you reflect on what you see, you will begin to have a deeper understanding of yourself.

As you review the patterns of your past, you may become acutely aware of what you did not get in your relationships. You may also become aware of sexual behaviors you engaged in that you didn't really enjoy. Or you may become aware of the kinds of attention that you did want but didn't receive.

It is important to acknowledge to yourself that filling out the chart is a major step in being honest about your sexual past. Give yourself credit for being willing to take that step. As with the Sexual History Lifeline, you can fill out the chart right in this book, in the *Awaken Your Sexuality Workbook*, or on a separate sheet of paper. Again, we urge you to *do the exercise*—don't just read about it. For the exercise to be meaningful, you need to fill out the spaces honestly, carefully thinking about your past relationships and their characteristics.

Naming your past in this systematic fashion is the key that unlocks your capacity for healing. Choices that you have made will be clearer, and times when you did not have a choice, or felt that you did not have a choice, will also be clearer. We cannot change the past, but we can change how we feel about it in the present, and we can change how we make decisions going forward.

Instructions for the Relationship History Chart

Across the top of the chart are spaces for the names of people with whom you remember having sexual relationships. You will make the call about what qualifies as a "relationship." (We suggest that if you had feelings about a person, even if they didn't return the feelings, it is best to include them.)

If there are sexual relationships you have trouble remembering because of your substance use or trauma symptoms, do not worry about trying to recall them. Work with the memories that are available to you. If you are currently in a relationship that has sexual expectations, even if you are avoiding sexual connection, put that person's name in the last (most recent) space.

In the other cells of the chart, you will fill in:

1. **Characteristics of the person.** List the words that best describe the person emotionally. Paint a descriptive picture of the person. Examples of words to describe the person might include *cold*, *warm*, *indirect*, *present*, *distant*, *affectionate*, *mean*, *caring*, *gentle*, *loyal*, *insecure*, *honest*, *reliable*, *sarcastic*, or *courageous*.

2. **Characteristics of the relationship.** Use words that best describe your interaction with this person—that is, how the relationship felt to you. Examples might include *caring*, *distant*, *fun*, *sympathetic*, *hopeless*, *warm*, *supportive*, *intense*, *uncommunicative*, *boring*, *deceitful*, *mutual*, *indifferent*, *critical*, *exciting*, *stable*, or *toxic*.

3. **Addictive behaviors.** Describe any problematic use of alcohol or other substances by you or your partner during the relationship, as well as other addictive/compulsive behaviors either of you might have engaged in.

4. **Sexual qualities of the relationship.** Pick words that best describe the sexual qualities of the relationship. You might consider whether the relationship was *mutual*, *passionate*, *one-sided*, *open*, *nonexistent*, *compulsive*,

accepting, shameful, tender, affectionate, routine, dutiful, adventurous, or *confusing*.

5. **Sexual likes and dislikes in the relationship.** Go through the sexual qualities of the relationship that you've just listed and sort them into two categories: those you liked and those you didn't. This is also the place to reflect on the sexual activities you engaged in and whether you generally liked or disliked them.

What to Look For

It is important to notice whether the words you use to describe the characteristics of the relationship are identical to the characteristics of the person you described. If they are, you can see the effect of your partner in that relationship. Where were you? What happened to the effect you had on the relationship? How did you express yourself in that relationship? What does this say about your power in the relationship? If you feel that your characteristics did not determine the character of the relationship at least in part, this is an important fact to notice.

You may also want to reflect on how often you have felt free to express yourself sexually in a relationship. How much of your sexual life has been determined by your partner's desires and preferences versus your own? Have you felt encouraged to ask for something new, to initiate sexual contact, to discuss sexual health practices like birth control and barriers for preventing the spread of STIs? Do you feel generally satisfied by the sexual connections you have had, or do you have one or two that really stand out? What were the qualities and characteristics of the sexual partnerships that brought you the most sexual satisfaction?

If the Relationship History Chart reveals uncomfortable patterns, know that you are not alone. Your courage and honesty will serve you well as you seek to create sexual relationships that are mutually fulfilling and supportive to your recovery.

Relationship History Chart

Name	1)	2)	3)	4)	5)
Characteristics of the person					
Characteristics of the relationship					
Addictive behaviors					
Sexual qualities of the relationship					
Sexual likes and dislikes in the relationship					

Living in the Present

Living in the present means that you are consciously aware of what is going on for you right now. You may say, "But of course I'm living in the present! Where else is there to live?" The fact is, however, that we spend most of our time either in the past, feeling uncomfortable about things we've already done, or in the future, worrying about, planning for, or trying to control events that haven't yet happened.

When we spend our time in the past, we carry our history around with us. We are burdened with expectations based on things that have happened to us, and we expect that these things will continue to happen to us. Or we may live in the future, like Rebecca, fantasizing each new relationship to a depressing conclusion before it even begins.

The realization that we have spent the better part of our lives ideating about the past or future can be disturbing. We've lost a lot of time and experience. But no matter how much of your life you've spent elsewhere, you can learn to live in the present, and you can reclaim your past without having to reexperience it. When you live in the present, you will reconnect with more of yourself.

Your Observer Self

Perhaps the best way to learn to live in the present is to allow your observer self into your consciousness. The *observer self* is a phrase used by mindfulness teachers and therapists to acknowledge a nonjudgmental part of you who acts as a witness to the events of your life. The observer self can look at how you feel and act and know that particular actions and feelings are not your total self. The observer self is a mirror in which you can look at your own behaviors and actions without judgment.

If you have spent many years in guilt and shame, you may not believe this aspect of yourself exists. But it does, and you can develop it.

Developing your observer self is different from dissociating from your body and feelings. Observing is not the same as stepping outside of yourself to avoid facing yourself. Observing is not the same as using the defense mechanism of abandoning yourself because it's too painful to be present. What your observer self does is provide you with a quiet place from which to view your own behavior with reflection and acceptance. Your observer self loves you unconditionally, no matter what.

Allowing your observer self to be with you on a daily basis will enable you to notice, for example, that you are having sex with a partner who does not seem interested in cultivating your pleasure. Your observer self can help you notice that the meeting you have been going to feels exciting because you are attracted to someone in the room. Your observer self might recognize a partner's behavior as similar to one of your parents'. Your observer self does not judge these realities, but simply brings them to your attention so that you can choose how to work with them. Your observer self is rooting for you.

A Daily Inventory

Your observer self helps you stay in the present. Staying in the present in relation to your sexuality and noticing what you are doing can be real work, but it is work that pays off as you become able to choose your sexual behavior rather than simply acting out unconscious patterns.

Taking a daily inventory can help this process. Writing things down in a journal can be especially helpful, because it allows you to review your progress.

For example, each night before you go to bed, you might ask yourself the following questions: Did I feel sexual/attractive/interested in sexuality today? How did I express this? You will soon find that it gets easier to recognize your feelings and to focus on their place in your life.

See the *Awaken Your Sexuality Workbook* for more journaling prompts. Write down how the journaling makes you feel too. Your feelings will change as you get accustomed to paying attention to and writing about your sexuality.

Another discovery that may emerge is the realization that you are a combination of the thoughts and feelings and experiences that have accumulated throughout your life. You may recognize that you still react like a child or adolescent in some situations. As you observe yourself, you may begin to recognize the inner child, the critical self, the shamed self, the romantic self, the workaday self, the mature adult self—all the different parts of yourself. You can begin to question the attitudes and beliefs that control the different aspects of yourself. Then you can begin to consciously choose which stance you will take in any given circumstance.

Partner selection involves choices. Understanding the influence of our past relationships is the first step. Seeing how and where they continue to affect us is the second. Realizing that we have choices about whom to select in the present and future is part of the awakening experience.

> National Domestic Violence Hotline:
> 1-800-799-SAFE (7233) or 1-800-787-3224 (TTY)
>
> ---
>
> Rape, Abuse & Incest National Network (RAINN)
> Sexual Assault Hotline: 1-800-656-HOPE (4673)

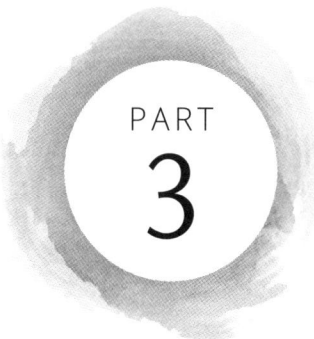

PART

3

The Power of Choice: Ongoing Recovery

The transition between early and ongoing recovery is marked by a feeling of reconnection with your inner observer self, that wise and nonjudgmental part of yourself from whom you have been estranged for so long. As you move into ongoing recovery, a stage that you will explore for the rest of your life, this connection with your observer self allows you to tackle deeper issues that were too overwhelming to handle earlier.

As you delve deeper, you will become aware of how guilt and shame have restricted your sexual energy and left you avoidant or compulsive, and therefore less able to choose the forms of sexual experience that resonate most with your inner self.

Many people find that their relationship issues rise to the surface after some period of recovery. This can be discouraging at first, but ultimately it is a sign that you are becoming more aware of how you feel and what you want. The issues can become clear because some space has been made for them. This is uncomfortable, but it does not mean you are doing anything wrong. On the contrary, you are in a new place, with new challenges. You have arrived at a new bend on the upward spiral.

In ongoing recovery, you will move toward healing the pain of prior sexual issues and dissolving your shame. When you are able to recognize and move through painful memories and feelings, you will discover your core of power.

Building a foundation of honesty is an essential element in early recovery. As you continue to build on this foundation in ongoing recovery, you will begin the major task of reclaiming your sense of empowerment. This will allow you to create a healthy, fulfilling sexual life, on your own terms.

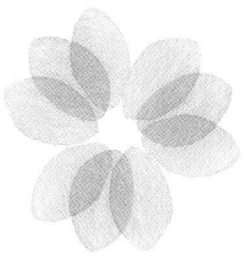

CHAPTER 8

Choosing a New Sexual Life

It is hard to describe to someone who has not
experienced it, what it is for a body to open, but
it is just as holy as falling before the pulpit and
as righteous as a riot. It is the breaking of what
binds. It is undoing so that we can become.

Prentis Hemphill, *What It Takes to Heal:*
How Transforming Ourselves Can Change the World

The journey of sexual recovery is developmental. You must walk down the path of early recovery before you can turn the corner into ongoing recovery. Yet each person creates their own unique version of that path, tackling these stages in their own way, doing inner work or taking outer actions as the need arises and issues present themselves.

Remember that the process of sexual awakening and recovering can take the form of an upward spiral (see Figure 1 on page 85). As you pass through one stage, and then another and another, you will revisit the same issues but on higher levels of understanding and work. Where first you needed the most basic definitions, now you also see the subtleties. Life seems to present the same issues over and over again. But when you are working on your recovery, you will see these issues with a new sense of depth and complexity. Progress means moving to another level of self-exploration, not "fixing" yourself or getting rid of a particular issue once and for all. A familiar situation arises, and rather than do what you've always done, you see more than one way to proceed. This is a key achievement!

The Twelve Step slogan "Progress, not perfection" is helpful for the process of sexual recovery. Your goal in sexual recovery is not to become a perfect lover but to become increasingly aware of the role sexuality plays in your life. You want to grow in your ability to recognize your sexual feelings and act on them. In that process, you will come to accept yourself as human. This means sometimes you shut down when you want to be open; sometimes you make inappropriate sexual demands on those you love; sometimes you miss opportunities to express caring through sexual touch; sometimes you are silent when you want to say no; sometimes you panic when everything seems fine.

As you move up the spiral to greater understanding, you will also begin to notice the times you are truly present for yourself and your partner, the times you treat your body and the bodies of those you touch with respect and love, the times you simply love yourself for being you, the times when you experience unexpected pleasures.

Sexual recovery is not a calm ocean that you sail over like a stately ocean liner. You will still have your ups and downs. But in recovery, you have more access to hope. You know that you can change your sexual patterns, because you already have. The hopelessness of feeling out of control is no longer your constant state of being. As you gain hope, you also begin to gain personal power.

The Power to Change

For many people in recovery, the phrase *powerless over alcohol* will be deeply familiar. It is a foundational concept in AA, and millions have been helped by it. Co-author Stephanie wrote in *A Woman's Way Through the Twelve Steps* that for her, "admitting my powerlessness over alcohol gave me a sense of relief and reassurance." The understanding that life has become unmanageable, however many times we may need to revisit the feeling, is a key component of becoming truthful with ourselves about our experience.

However, the feeling of powerlessness is also a painful feature of trauma. This means that "admitting" powerlessness over trauma symptoms may not feel clarifying; it may feel confusing or even demeaning. When someone exerted power over you in a way that caused you harm, you were not empowered to stop the harm in the moment. If you have survived a trauma such as a car accident, natural disaster, incarceration, or military deployment to a combat zone, powerlessness is a nightmarish feature of the experience. This is also true for people who have survived the effects of structural injustices such as sexism, racism, homophobia, transphobia, ableism, and the myriad ways marginalization can cause us harm. When the world you were born into was not built for you to thrive in it, powerlessness can be a feature of everyday life.

Emphasizing powerlessness can make a person with a trauma history feel like nothing has changed from when they were in danger. Studies show that out-of-control behaviors, including substance use disorders, eating disorders, and other addictions, increase along with trauma symptoms. When we survive a trauma, we may use drugs, alcohol, sex, food, or any other behavior to try to control the emotions and sensations that arise in us. In other words, many addictions begin as a way for us to help ourselves through trauma symptoms—including the experience of being a woman or gender-diverse person in a patriarchal society. Ultimately, we may find that the substance or behavior becomes its own problem, and recognizing that, we may be forced back into painful memories and feelings of being out of control. This can be a demoralizing downward spiral.

Ironically, when we recognize that our behavior or our lives are out of control, we can actually begin the process of regaining personal power. Healing from trauma requires that we feel empowered to make choices, not forced to do things. Healing from addiction may require that we push ourselves to quit doing something we've loved doing. We may have to rise to the challenge of going to a group meeting with people we've never met, or overcome our reticence and talk about our feelings to a therapist. There is a balance of challenge and safety we have to find.

The fear of feeling forced to do things can keep trauma survivors feeling stuck and discouraged about their capacity to make changes in their lives. It is a complication, but it is not an impossible obstacle. You will likely need to regularly tap into something larger than yourself and receive help and support to navigate the tension. Your ability to make choices, give consent freely, and affirm what you want are all foundational for your sexual recovery.

For Nova, a revelation came one day when she did not want to host the recovery meeting she had started for her sex-working community. She felt exhausted, having helped someone through a crisis the night before. During a morning call with a friend, Nova felt ashamed for not wanting to run the meeting—she valued service and feared being seen as "selfish." Her friend told her it was perfectly okay to take the day off and ask someone else to host.

"In fact," her friend said, "your sobriety probably will feel easier to maintain today if you rest." Nova recognized the signs of unmanageability in others' lives faster than in her own. She believed that she should be stronger, more capable, and more resilient than the people she was helping. But then she realized: The only reason she was able to help others was because she consistently received support, rest, camaraderie, friendship, and care. The power to change her own life was not derived from her constant activity or self-sacrifice, but from her interconnectedness.

"I still needed some permission to rest," Nova recounted later. "I am working on learning to give that permission to myself."

Pay attention to the interplay between your personal power to effect change in yourself and the world around you, and the larger collective power of the family, friend groups, and movements you are part of. When you feel powerless, you can seek support. When you feel powerful, you can offer strength and support to yourself and others. An ebb and flow is to be expected.

Money, Social Influence, and Sex

The statistics are staggering: Women are still paid less than men at every education and income level. The gap is smallest among low-wage workers (due in part to there being a minimum wage), but for middle-income workers, the gap is nearly 15 percent, and it widens to over 22 percent for earners in the ninetieth percentile. Black and Hispanic women experience the largest pay gaps—even when education, experience, and regional economic conditions are factored in.[1]

Queer people, especially bisexual and lesbian cisgender women, transgender women, and nonbinary people, are more likely to live in poverty than heterosexual women or men. Housing and employment discrimination affects LGBTQ+ people at higher rates. This also means that LGBTQ+ people are less likely to receive high-quality health benefits via employment, which can affect recovery outcomes. These economic injustices lead many queer women, trans women, and nonbinary and gender-expansive people to rely on co-living, often with partners, to make ends meet, especially if they are parents.

Comparisons of women and men after divorce consistently show larger drops in financial well-being for women. This lack of economic power leads women to stay in marriages that no longer fulfill them sexually or emotionally, or to stay with men who are violent and abusive. Even relatively financially stable middle-class single mothers find it difficult to afford childcare while they work, and this influences their relationship decisions.

The major takeaway here is that our economic options mold and influence our sexual relationship decisions. We are not choosing partners in an ideal world of freedom and endless possibilities; we are engaging with real people while we all navigate prejudiced systems.

Given this reality, the more you know your own body, feelings, and desires, the more empowered you can be to advocate for the sexual life you want, regardless of your financial situation. You, caring for your body and developing an understanding of your own sexual feelings, are remaining as powerfully grounded in your own choices as is possible.

Trading Sex for Something Else

There may be times in our lives when making sexual choices is more an act of survival than of pleasure. The choice to trade sex for safety, drugs, a place to sleep, money, acceptance, the promise of a promotion, or anything else of value appears in many forms and at many different moments in our lives. It is not an uncommon experience for sex to become a commodity we can barter with.

Sexual recovery involves making these experiences conscious, and understanding when you feel empowered to choose how you engage sexually with others, and when you don't—or haven't. Sometimes our choices change drastically when we become more aware of our power to choose. Sometimes we are engaged in the same behaviors, but how we feel about them changes.

When Nova first began working in a strip club, she was aware that she would be selling a sexual performance. She was comfortable showing her body and being in contact with men and women customers, and she did not feel ashamed of her work. She was connected to several sex workers' rights groups online and considered herself part of a political movement. Nova believed that consenting adults should have the right to private sexual transactions. When she started a recovery group for sex workers, she knew that it would feel much safer for her to talk about her work with people who had a similar life experience. Although she did not primarily work as an escort or companion, she had spent many nights with customers—partying, getting high, having sex. She sometimes would receive cash gifts for her time.

When Nova got sober, some of these sources of extra income dried up. She still did well dancing at her club, so she was able to stay financially stable, and slowly she built a clientele who were supportive of her sobriety. When she began addressing her disordered eating and decided to be celibate for a time, she encountered some more challenges—her management at the club commented when she gained weight, for instance.

Nova began to brainstorm other ways to use her skills to bring in income, like teaching pole dancing classes and monetizing a YouTube channel with her popular videos. Her community was instrumental in supporting Nova through the challenges she faced. They met online every week and helped each other maintain their commitments to their recovery. One issue many of them faced was the pressure they felt they were under to drink and do drugs with their clients. Some felt that it was easier just to say yes, even if it undermined their sobriety. Nova knew that wouldn't have worked for her.

"First, I really had to commit to not using alcohol and drugs of any kind. I wasn't a casual user; I was definitely addicted to meth, and alcohol often led to me using. So I just needed to back off completely. But also, I don't think being high made it easier to do sex work," Nova told her peer group. "I think I would have said it did at the time, but really it made it harder. I had horrible hangovers all the time. I was embarrassed about stuff I'd said and done. I'd black out and not remember if I'd negotiated properly with a customer. Being high made me sloppy. It also kept me from knowing myself and what my real boundaries were."

"But isn't it harder to go in to work now?" a friend in the group asked.

Nova considered how to answer the question. "I'm more present in my body, and so I have to say no more often now, which is scary, because what if the customer gets mad, or I don't get paid? But I still have clients because there are plenty of people who enjoy being with me as I am. I have clearer boundaries, which feels good to me. I go to bed feeling good about myself, and I wake up knowing what happened. There's nothing I would trade for that peace of mind."

For Nova, it was possible to trade her sexual attention for money without feeling exploited, demeaned, or disempowered overall. Her experience is not uncommon, although every person who enters sex work of any kind—legal or illegal, in person or online, on or off camera—will be faced with complex negotiations around personal power and boundaries. The criminalization of some forms of sex work affects every choice.

Ash, like Nova, had many sexual experiences that revolved around drugs and monetary support. Unlike Nova, Ash did not use the term *sex work* for these trades. Considering the age differences and exploitative nature of many of Ash's early sexual experiences, what happened to them would have met the criteria for human trafficking. But that term didn't feel right to Ash, either.

When speaking about their sexual experiences as a young person, Ash often used the word *trade*. "I traded sex for heroin and a place to sleep," or "I traded sex for an overnight pass out of the group home," or "I had sex so the manager would look the other way when I came to work late." For Ash, these trades all had material goals in mind. Some of the experiences were traumatic, but many of them were not.

Trading sex was part of Ash's story, part of how they survived after childhood sexual abuse and through addiction, homelessness, and involvement with the criminal legal system. It was difficult for Ash to speak about these experiences at first, but eventually they discovered that their honesty about their life allowed others to feel welcome to speak openly about their own experiences. As Ash progressed in their recovery, they were able to make more conscious choices about their sexual body. They felt more empowered, in large part because they were holding a job and stabilizing financially.

It is very common for women, especially heterosexual women, to stay with partners they no longer love for the sake of economic support. This may actually be one of the more common forms of sexual trade in our society today. It is not the same as engaging in sex work, in large part because it is not stigmatized or criminalized. But it is still a form of trade. This type of trade is a major piece of co-author Stephanie's story.

Stephanie had been married to her ex-husband for thirteen years. After one year of sobriety, she got divorced and got custody of their children.

Stephanie recalls, "I got married in the middle of graduate school, partly because of family pressure, partly to keep up with my younger sister, who'd gotten married the summer before, and partly because I'd never been on my own. My parents had paid my way through school, and I knew I couldn't support myself in the same style my family had provided.

"My husband was tall and handsome, a few years older than me, already financially established, and ready to settle down with a wife and family. He was just the kind of man my family wanted for me. He had a good job, he was successful, he liked traveling and going to good restaurants, he dressed well, he'd buy us a safe and quiet house in the suburbs. It all seemed perfect.

"Of course, what no one knew was that I'd been drinking heavily since my freshman year in college. I was in a sorority, and drinking was a perfectly socially acceptable party activity. But I'd been having blackouts since the beginning. Being married was ideal for me in terms of drinking. I felt safe; I could drink at home from the cocktail hour on without worrying about what would happen. Even though I continued to have blackouts, I thought everyone who drank forgot things.

"The real problem was that within a month of getting married, I knew I'd made a mistake. My husband and I just weren't compatible emotionally, politically, or sexually, and as a result, we fought often.

"So there I was in the suburbs drinking wine at lunch and then drinking from the cocktail hour until bedtime. I knew I was unhappy, but I wasn't able to face it. Then, of course, I got pregnant. More than once.

"Having those babies to look after pretty much destroyed any possibility that I'd leave the marriage. Sure, I knew I wasn't really there for my children, especially at night. I put them to bed as early as I could, completely dependent upon my husband to handle nighttime requests from the children. I knew if we were divorced and something happened, I would not be in any shape to function. I was too high to deal with any problems by eight or nine at night. I was afraid. I knew that as long as I was drinking like that, I couldn't count on myself to respond in a crisis.

"My husband never expressed any unhappiness with the marriage. I was attractive, well dressed, and socially adept, and other people thought I was a good mother. I looked good on the outside and was the kind of wife that he wanted. I helped him have the kind of life he wanted to live.

"But inside, things weren't so great. Our relationship continued to deteriorate, and our verbal fights got really mean and vindictive. I knew I wasn't happy and was just staying with him because I was afraid that without him I couldn't take care of the children. I constantly threatened to leave, but never once followed through.

"I remember attending a luncheon in the mid-seventies where Gloria Steinem and Phyllis Chesler were the speakers. Part of their presentation talked about women in marriages where the love was lost but they stayed for financial security. That it was a trade-off. I said to my friend at lunch that if I believed them, I needed to get a divorce. Instead, I went home and got drunk.

"Finally, I 'hit my bottom,' called up AA, and went to a meeting. I got a sponsor and stayed sober with only one slip. But I knew that I needed to leave the marriage; I'd never really been there emotionally, even at the beginning. I told my husband that they suggested in AA not to make any big changes during the first year, but that once the year was up, I was going out the door. I knew then that I could take care of the kids myself, even if it was hard. I wasn't drunk anymore at night; now I could be responsible.

"Luckily, I received some assets in the divorce settlement, and my parents were there as a backup if needed. I look back now and see how many years I stayed in a marriage because I couldn't stop drinking and was afraid of not having enough money."

Like all who divorce, Stephanie had to work to put her life back together. She needed to learn to parent alone and to meet her own needs directly and without alcohol. At first, she was surprised that her graduate degree in social work did not prepare her for work in the addiction field because she didn't have three years of recovery.

Stephanie learned to feel compassion for herself during those years. She had exchanged her ability to be a "good" wife for the freedom to be able to drink. In recovery, she went back to school to obtain a PhD, volunteered in a treatment program, and started a process of discovering who she really was sexually.

Stephanie knew it was difficult and scary to live an honest life. She knew how long it took her to make a move, and she was especially understanding with the women who came into treatment. She knew about the struggles and the trade-offs that had to be worked through in order to live honestly.

Respecting Hopelessness

The path of ongoing recovery is not linear. On an upward spiral, you may have some of the same issues for the rest of your life, but your relationship to those issues changes. Sometimes a sexual issue is in the foreground, moves to the background, then comes back again.

It would be lovely if we could promise that once you begin investigating your sexual feelings and making peace with your body, you will feel better and better each day. But that would be dishonest. For many people, sexual recovery brings painful challenges because it involves facing trauma without the numbing effect of their addictions.

People can become extremely fearful about sex without alcohol or other substances. They may feel awkward, unsure of themselves, or frustrated about how difficult it seems to get close to people without the "bonding" that happens while drinking or using together. During recovery from problem use of a substance, disordered eating, or other compulsive behavior, sexual joy may not be available at first. When it all seems too, too hard and the future is fearsome, hopelessness may take us over. This is a powerful experience and requires care and attention to move through.

Respecting hopelessness means recognizing and allowing the feeling to enter, and in doing so, feeling it fully, *without taking self-harming action*. In fact, the more gently and tenderly we can treat ourselves in the face of it, the more swiftly hopelessness will transform into something else. That something else only needs to be a sliver of light, a crack in the wall of pain.

When co-author Vanessa was in early recovery, they felt a crushing shame about every horrible choice they had ever made and every painful experience they had survived. Without drugs to numb the feelings, Vanessa began to feel hopeless about ever being well. Their life partnership had ended dramatically, they were struggling to get work and feared losing their housing, they were lonely and exhausted from years of PTSD symptoms: panic attacks, trouble with intimate touch, repeated illnesses, and chronic pain. It all seemed impossible to overcome.

Then Vanessa had an older mentor and friend who said something surprising. She told Vanessa, "Go into that hopelessness. Let hopelessness put you on the floor. Breathe hopelessness. Make hopelessness welcome in your family of feelings."

When Vanessa allowed the feeling of hopelessness to fully bloom, it was truly terrible. Vanessa entered a state of suicidal ideation. This was only safe to do because they weren't alone with their feelings; they had guidance and love from someone who had been there before. The mentor then gently asked: "Do you want to stop being alive? Or do you just want the pain to end?"

This became a turning point. Realizing that what they most wanted was for the pain to end, Vanessa was able to reach out to more people for help. They began the long process of listening to, attending to, and mending the sources of their pain.

Vanessa remembers, "I thought I'd rather be high than be hopeless. I was always fighting for the next save—I'm going to save my relationship by sacrificing myself just a little more. I'm going to save my loved one from their own addiction. I'm going to save my spot in my program, even though I'm not well enough to learn. I thought if I let hopelessness arrive, it would kill me. But instead, hopelessness was the place from which I could really face that I needed change.

"Hopelessness was my way of accepting that I had failed—even if I'd bailed out some water, I hadn't yet changed the reality: The ship of my life was sinking. My years-long life partnership was over, and I wasn't sure I'd ever recover from that loss. I certainly couldn't imagine feeling love or loved again. The hopelessness of that heartache was the opening to my grief, and when I started really grieving, I was astounded to find a tiny part of me that wanted to live on, to see what happened next."

Hopelessness is a response to pain that seems intractable. It can creep in after years of recovery work, on a bad day, on the heels of a disappointment, as a companion to a relapse, or hiding in a hurtful conversation. It sounds like "I can't do this," "I don't want to do this anymore," "I should feel better by now," and "It never ends."

Working now as a death doula, a person who supports the dying and their loved ones, Vanessa is in contact with true, end-of-the-line, intractable suffering and disease. When someone is dying, people often tell them, "Don't give up, don't lose hope." But sometimes, acknowledging that the end of life is near is the opposite of hopelessness. Death is a truth for all of us, and accepting its inevitability need not be the same thing as "giving up." It can be a freedom and a place where true feeling emerges.

People living with terminal illness, who are preparing for their own deaths, are sometimes filled with terror at the unknown. But terror, hopelessness, and despair are only part of the experience. Usually there is also tenderness, reverence for life, and a blazing love that they want to make sure to communicate to the people closest to them.

When we hit a wall of hopelessness, we are under a delusion that nothing will change. In fact, change comes whether we create it consciously or not. Time does not stop with our pain, and change is inevitable. Hopelessness is an indication that we are walking into our darker places and fearing that we may stay there.

If hopelessness visits you in your recovery process, ask someone you trust to sit alongside you as you let it roll through. If it persists and becomes an ongoing threat to your mental or physical health, you can call in more reinforcements: inpatient or outpatient programs, recovery groups, sponsors, accountability partners, professional therapists, loved ones, and so on. Respecting hopelessness means allowing it, but also moving through it. We feel, rest, and then try again tomorrow.

Suicide and Crisis Lifeline: Call or text 988

The Courage to Act

Recovery of any kind is about wanting to change. Sexual recovery is about self-empowerment, pleasure, connection, and intimacy. We must make the decision to explore and identify choices, to become aware of our options. As you gain awareness and expand your capacity to meet your own needs, you can start to enlarge your capacity to act intentionally rather than react instinctively. You increase your personal power as you increase your capacity to produce change in your own life, and as you connect with other people on a similar path, you can contribute more to your community and collectives.

In our society, *power* has often meant *power over*: the ability to dominate and control others. Historically, that power has been enforced by violence. Americans today have inherited an understanding of power that was forged in colonialism, slavery, patriarchal control of women, land theft, and genocidal wars against Indigenous peoples. American democratic control of the government, however different it may have seemed from the divine right of kings, was yet reserved for a small number of white men, many of whom were enslavers. The power of "the people" was reserved for a small number of people.

Women, nonbinary people, and gender-expansive people are no strangers to the effects of this type of power. In addition to the structural barriers we face, power imbalances are often reflected in families and exhibited in intimate partner violence. Any of us are capable of bullying those with less power than us, exerting our will over others without their consent. We all live in a complex and dynamic set of systems—workplaces, schools, religious institutions, medical and mental health institutions, criminal and civil legal systems, and more—which affect and influence our experience of the hierarchies of power.

At the same time as *power over* seeks to dominate and control, there have always been those looking to build a different form of power, what many now call *power with*. This is collective and personal power based in mutuality, empathy, care, and respect. It asks us to take responsibility for our own actions. It asks us to approach other people with curiosity and to seek connection. Creating power with others means we build the capacity to change our lives together, because of each other, not in spite of each other. This type of power is love in action.

When you devote yourself to your own recovery from addiction and trauma, you may initially feel as if you are doing much of the work alone, but the truth is you are joining millions of other people who are trying to get better, just like you. When you commit to your sexual well-being, the same is true. Because sexuality is such a foundational part of who we are as humans (including those times when we are not sexually active or desirous), your curiosity and care for your sexual self can connect you to something much larger than you.

It takes immense courage, but you can take responsibility for where you are now. You can act in accordance with your values. You can make amends where appropriate and learn to respond consciously as new sexual situations happen. You can recognize that you may need more sexual education, and seek out the information you need. You can identify that you have some choices about how your sexual life unfolds, and that you can exercise them. You can accept your power to respond differently to events over which you may have no control.

The path of growth, the upward spiral, is always a path that requires renewed choice on a daily basis. We grow in our ability to choose recovery and to choose a conscious path of self-empowerment. It is never easy or quick. Taking a step at a time, and allowing others to support those steps of growth, produces its own reward in a sense of well-being and a growing hope of the possibility of expansion.

○ ○ ○

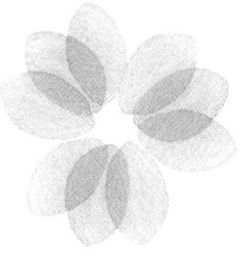

CHAPTER 9

Choosing Personal Power

Of what have I ever been afraid? To question or to speak as I believed could have meant pain, or death. But we all hurt in so many different ways, all the time, and the pain will either change or end. . . . And I began to recognize a source of power within myself that comes from the knowledge that, while it is most desirable not to be afraid, learning to put fear into a perspective gives me great strength. My silences had not protected me. Your silence will not protect you.

———

Audre Lorde, *Sister Outsider:
Essays and Speeches*

Those of us in recovery keep ourselves from using our personal power in many ways, but three are most common: by living in constant self-punishment for our destructive behavior in the past, by taking blame or inappropriate responsibility for abuse we endured, and by identifying with our shame more than our curiosity or pleasure.

When you choose to make changes in these areas, more empowerment, presence, and connection become possible. Sexuality can become creative, a source of energy and interest, rather than a place of fear or numbness. This is where you feel empowered to choose and connect. It is where your personal power is cultivated, and your pleasure is welcome. It takes time, but these changes are possible. You will need to develop your self-compassion.

Guilt, Shame, and Self-Compassion

Guilt can have a positive function: It is a sign that we care about others' feelings, that we understand our own values, and that our behavior needs a course correction. We experience guilt when we feel that we have violated our own values, when we feel we have done something that goes against who we think we are or should be. Guilt also accompanies feelings of regret and remorse about something we have done. Most often we feel guilty about something we have done to someone else. When we cause harm to someone, guilt tells us we wish we hadn't.

Once we have made our apologies, if they are possible and do not cause further harm, and take responsibility for our behavior, guilt should begin to recede. Our ability to feel remorse for our actions is crucial to human relationships. It can also spring up when we are reminded of harm we have caused in the past. A pang of guilt about something we did in the past is a normal part of being a social human. It is a sign we want to take responsibility for our actions.

However, when we feel persistent, overwhelming guilt, we may struggle to live in the present because we are stuck on something unresolved that we regret having done in the past. It is very common for women in recovery to be heavily burdened with guilt related to sexual issues. A feature of rape culture is that women internalize the blame and feel guilty for experiences that we did not cause. This is especially true for survivors of sexual assault who knew their attacker, who are in community or family with the person or people who harmed them.

Those who live with addiction have an added burden. Women, nonbinary people, and gender-expansive people with addiction are more stigmatized than men. It is common to internalize that stigma and subsequently feel shame for being addicted and shame for the sexual events that occurred during that time.

Guilt that persists, which becomes a heavier and heavier burden as time goes on, is an exhaustingly painful experience. For many people, this type of guilt morphs from "I am sorry for what I have done" into something more all-encompassing: "I am ashamed of who I am." If guilt is about what we have done, then shame is about who we believe we are. Shame can become a pervasive and constant feature of our emotional life.

Shame enters through all levels of our experience, including our families, our communities, and our larger society. Shame is a consequence of personal events, such as being told there is something wrong with you by someone you trust. It is also a feature of systemic prejudice, which plays out in both large and small ways in virtually every school, place of worship, workplace, community, city, county, and so on.

In a country built on the belief that white skin made a person superior, children of color absorb shaming experiences and grow up enduring shame's constricting and restricting influence. Queer and trans children absorb shame from their environments. People in bigger bodies, disabled people, neurodivergent people, poor people, and many more are contending with the way shame from American culture becomes part of our identities.

Politically, a response to the shame doled out by our culture is often framed as "pride," because pride feels like the opposite of shame. And it is a beautiful experience to be among people who feel proud of who they are. But pride doesn't always feel like the appropriate response for trauma survivors or those who live with addictions.

Many survivors of childhood sexual abuse, for example, have a complex relationship with feeling proud of who they are. Like Ash often says to their peer counseling clients: "Some days, I'm so proud of making it this far, of choosing to be alive, and I want everyone to know that I've survived all kinds of odds. Other days, I just want to be normal and not think about any of it." Sometimes, Ash does not want to be defined only by what they have survived.

Shame is a cruel and slippery feature of surviving trauma, abuse, and addiction. We may know that we didn't want to be hurt, or to cause harm, but we still feel that we are no good at our very core. This feeling is so horrifying, so burdensome, that we become secretive about our shame. We don't want anyone to know how bad we are. There is sometimes another twist: We feel we are supposed to be able to overcome shame simply and quickly. Therefore, when shame persists, we feel shame about our shame, as in, we become ashamed that we couldn't get better faster.

As solid and impervious as shame may feel, you can eventually dissolve it. If pride in who you are feels far away, because of how much guilt and shame you still carry, the work of self-compassion is the way to lighten your load. Self-compassion is an ongoing practice, a crucial part of recovery. Now, as we move along the upward spiral of recovery and healing, we will enrich our understanding of it.

You have already begun the work of addressing your shame by looking into your past and telling yourself the truth about your sexual life so far. We now ask you to actively develop a robust sense of self-compassion. Self-compassion and the cultivation of pleasure and intimacy go hand in hand.

Shame Drains Your Power; Self-Compassion Restores It

Shameful feelings can be triggered by internal or external experiences. Ongoing recovery is about empowerment, the ability to feel your personal power and take action. Healing your sense of shame is basic to your empowerment.

Shame immobilizes you and drains away your power. You may feel that you have no energy, no hope, no sense of the possibility of movement. In this way, shame becomes a vicious circle. The more ashamed you feel, the more you are robbed of your initiative. You don't move out into the world as much, and therefore you have fewer positive, affirming experiences.

Taking a careful look at the source of shame in your life is an important step toward becoming more self-compassionate. You will certainly find that you have no control over many things. You may have internalized shame about any number of aspects of yourself, such as your gender, race, ethnicity, or cultural background, where you grew up, what your body looks like, and your sexual orientation.

Some things about you can change, and others can't. Shame does not know the difference. It will show up to hurt you about parts of you that are completely unchangeable. But the variety we all embody is what gives life its rich complexity! If you are in touch with your wise inner observer self, you will know that there does not need to be shame attached to any part of who you are. It is the prejudice of the world around you that is the problem.

Reducing the influence of your shaming experiences is a long-term process. There is no easy cure or quick fix. Effecting such change takes time. Be patient with yourself as you move through this process.

Remember that shame existed before you were born, and you learned about it before you could speak. Parents changing a diaper swat their child's hand away from their own genitals, sending a clear message: "Touching yourself is bad." Young children are prone to simplifying messages like these, and soon they learn: "I'm bad." Undoing the grip shame has on you will not happen overnight. The self-compassion you develop will help you every time shame resurfaces.

EXERCISE

Working with *Should*

One way that shame drains our power is by constantly berating us. Internally, you can begin to hear the voice of shame whenever you hear the word *should*.

There are definitely some *shoulds* in our lives that are helpful and do not need to make us feel ashamed. For example: "If I want to pick up the kids on time, I should leave in five minutes."

Or maybe "I'm feeling lonely today; I should look at my list of people I can call and try one of them." There's also "It was extremely stressful to me to set that boundary with my partner. I should pay attention to my body and support myself."

But that's not how most of us use *should*. We use it instead to tell ourselves we are wrong, broken, and lacking. See if any of the following statements feel familiar:

- It's been years since my trauma happened. I should be over it by now.
- My sexual assault wasn't really violent, so I shouldn't have so much trouble with sex.
- I should be more successful.
- I should be stronger, smarter, and more assertive in social situations.
- My partner should find someone less broken than me.
- I shouldn't have done [that substance, that behavior], so everything that happened to me is my fault.
- I should want more/less sex.

Make your own list of shaming *should* statements, from three to five sentences. Now go back and write down a response to each, from the perspective of your observer self. Remember, this is the part of you that loves you unconditionally, roots for you, and genuinely wants you to feel well, happy, connected to your sexuality, and safe. For example, in response to the first statement above, "It's been years since my trauma happened; I should be over it by now," the writer's observer self might suggest:

> It's understandable that I get frustrated and impatient when I experience symptoms. Trauma healing can be unpredictable, and I can recognize when I need extra support. When I experience symptoms, I can use my resources to support me. I commit to caring for myself no matter what.

This dialogue begins as a writing exercise (see the *Awaken Your Sexuality Workbook* for more opportunity to practice) and can eventually become something you do automatically when you identify the shaming voice inside. Rather than allowing shame to bully you, you can gently reaffirm your inherent worth and dignity, identify resources that can support you in your feelings, and set the intention to care for yourself, no matter what.

Life After Sexual Trauma

Despite the many ways we can compartmentalize, cut off, ignore, or repress our sexual feelings, our sexuality does not exist in isolation from the rest of us. If we have been hurt sexually, we will be affected. Every person who experiences sexual trauma is unique in their experience. At the same time, there are some patterns to recognize in the way sexual trauma can happen, and what helps survivors of sexual trauma recover.

Researchers and people who create law and policy divide sexual trauma first by age: There is childhood sexual abuse (CSA) on one side of an eighteenth birthday, and sexual assault (SA) on the other. State laws differ in how they define rape, SA, CSA, sexual harassment, and other sexual offenses, like indecent exposure or statutory rape. In many states, SA and CSA encompass multiple acts, and so they are the terms we will use going forward. The main reason to use SA over other terms is to offer survivors an umbrella term that does not define exactly the nature of their experience and leaves room for each person's story to emerge at their choice, in their own time.

In addition to respecting every person's choice to name their experience, we would like to avoid reinforcing a strict hierarchy of harms—this attack was worse than that one—even though the criminal legal system does so. Sexual violation can occur at a distance or up close, online or in person, and it can be confusing, especially if it happened with someone you were attracted to, while you were intoxicated, during something you originally consented to, or if it is difficult to remember clearly.

It can be tempting to compare your experience to others, to measure the intensity of your suffering after sexual trauma. Rather than try to decide "how bad" your experience was based on the imagined or real experiences of others, we encourage you to use your feelings in the present as your guide. Like Roxane Gay wrote in *Not That Bad: Dispatches from Rape Culture*, "I finally reconciled my own past enough to realize that what I had endured was that bad, that what anyone has suffered is that bad."[1]

Whatever your lived experience, what matters is that you are honest with yourself about how you are doing, how you have been affected, and how you want to feel in your body, in your relationships, and in your sexuality. The work of recovery is different for everyone.

Sexual Assault in Rape Culture

Sexual assault (SA) is an ever-present possibility in women's lives. Most women are all too aware of this, and to some degree it limits how we live our daily lives. Most who identify as women are concerned about their physical safety and have places where they do not go alone, times they will not go outside, and situations they are careful to avoid. Few women can protect themselves so completely that they can disavow or completely ignore the risks attached to their gender.

The statistics vary depending on the source, but somewhere between one in six and one in four women experience SA in their lifetime. If we look just at trans women, the number jumps up to

50 percent to 66 percent.[2] While there are not currently statistics looking at the prevalence of SA for nonbinary individuals, those who identify under the umbrella of LGBTQ+ are at greater risk of violence than straight, cisgender women. This is a staggering amount of violence.

Rape culture is a term we use for the societal forces that normalize this level of violence and allow it to continue. It includes everything from a sudden, unexpected, unwanted kiss in a movie being framed as a "misunderstanding" to the laws we enact about sexual violence.

Until the latter half of the 1970s, it was not a crime in the United States for a man to force sexual intercourse on his wife. Marital rape was not recognized as a crime in all fifty states until 1993. According to the National Resource Center on Domestic Violence, about a third of women surveyed still reported just over a decade later to having "unwanted sex" with their partner.[3]

Today's "rape shield laws" are designed to protect victims of SA from inquiry into their prior sexual conduct—but why are they necessary? They are in place because for most of the twentieth century, criminal courts allowed a man accused of rape to defend himself by pointing to a woman's "unchaste reputation" or her "conduct that implied a lack of chastity."[4] In other words, "she asked for it" and "she deserved it" were viable defenses until very recently. It is no wonder this sexist logic still has so much power in our social world.

Historians draw explicit connections from current sexual violence law back to our country's history of chattel slavery and colonial war against Indigenous peoples. The way sexual assault victims of color have been harmed by the powerfully racist, sexist messages of rape culture are layered and long-standing, and these messages have, for centuries, been codified in the law. Sexual violence against enslaved women was not only commonplace; it was not a crime in most states where slavery was legal. The restriction of tribal authority and imposition of colonial government ensured that there would be little to no accountability for violence against Native women. While white women definitely have suffered under patriarchal laws, they also have been complicit in the harms caused against women of color for centuries.

The positive changes that are happening now as a result of organized efforts are real, but they are also quite recent. Male entitlement to use violence against women's bodies has been repeated and reinforced for hundreds of years. It would be nearly impossible *not* to internalize the messages of rape culture as a source of shame.

Women who fight against this oppression have to begin by feeling that we deserve to make decisions about our own bodies and lives. We have to band together and support each other in this belief, and we have to take action. This is why your integrity and self-compassion are so necessary. Integrity and self-compassion build the first step in your participation in a broader change for everyone.

If you experienced SA while you were drinking or using drugs, you probably blame yourself even more than you would if you had not been intoxicated. It is important to remind yourself that no circumstance justifies SA. Nothing about you, how you were dressed, how much you had to drink, or what you "didn't do to prevent it" has anything to do with SA. The violation of your sexual boundaries is the responsibility of the person who did the violating.

Thousands of people have been working to turn the tide on rape culture for decades, and there are changes happening. On college campuses all over the United States, administrations have adopted policies calling for "affirmative consent." An affirmative consent policy requires the people involved in a sexual act to give and receive verbal consent. A yes is a yes. The absence of a yes is actually a no.

Affirmative consent takes the notion that "no means no" a step further and challenges young people to communicate their interest and willingness to engage in sexual touch directly with each other. Whether these policies will protect people from SA has yet to be tested, but the discussions of what constitutes SA, and the importance of consent for all parties involved in a sexual interaction, are a move in the right direction.

Childhood Sexual Abuse

Many who experience SA are also survivors of CSA. Sexual abuse during childhood isn't limited to the specific acts of fondling and penetration. It occurs across a continuum, from invasion of sexual privacy to unwanted comments about your body, being kissed in a way that felt uncomfortable, being touched when you didn't want to be, and being pressured to have sexual contact you didn't want. You may have been sexually mistreated in a variety of ways that you didn't initially identify as sexual abuse. Yet those instances can greatly affect your current sexual feelings and experiences.

Ash had specific memories of CSA perpetrated by their step-father, but they also had suspicions that there may have been other men involved at other times. At first, they felt compelled to remember details, but ultimately, they had to accept that some of what happened to them may not be retrievable. A person does not need to have explicit memories of sexual abuse in childhood to have trouble with sexuality as an adult.

Identifying some family patterns from your childhood may help support you as you seek to build your self-compassion. Each of the following patterns can leave children more vulnerable to CSA from a teen or adult outside the family too.

Thinking back to where and how you grew up, see if any of the following might apply:

1. **Sexuality was totally repressed.** Family members/caregivers showed little or no affection and rarely touched, and the no-talk rule about sexuality was strictly enforced. Children in this environment learn about sex totally from peers, school, and other outside sources, and they often feel a great deal of shame about their sexuality.

2. **Sexuality was expressed only when a parent or other caregiving adult was drunk, high, or otherwise intoxicated.** For people who grew up with this dynamic, sexuality may seem humiliating and out of control, something to be totally avoided, or something they must always have strict control of. They may also repeat the pattern, expressing sexual feeling only when they are drinking or using.

3. **Sexuality was coupled with violence.** The only time a child saw their parent being sexual was after an argument or fight. The association between sexuality and violence can be difficult to unravel as a recovering adult. It is also common for sexuality to be associated with both substance use and violence.

4. **Sexual boundaries were not respected.** Children's changing needs for boundaries were not respected as they grew up. Caregivers may have touched without consent, made unwelcome comments, and been aggressive about their own "right" to act sexually in front of the children. It can be difficult to identify and establish boundaries later in life because they were not respected in childhood.

Giving Your Trauma Loving Attention

Healing is possible. Women in recovery deal with the effects of SA and CSA in various ways. Many sexual trauma survivors find that both group process and individual therapy are helpful. Group work with other survivors allows you to get to know and identify with others who have been through similar experiences. You will be able to feel at a much deeper level that you are not alone, that it is not all in your head, and that your reactions and feelings are shared by others.

Sexual trauma groups usually are led by skilled, licensed therapists who have experience working with people with trauma. Some groups are led by trained facilitators who are not therapists, and some peer groups share facilitation tasks. Groups vary in size and duration, and online or in-person format. It is affirming to bond with others who have had similar experiences. The release from isolation, secrecy, and shame can be liberating.

Individual trauma therapy is particularly good for understanding your present relationships, for exploring the effect SA or CSA is having on them, and for making the changes in your life that you are ready to make. Rape crisis centers and women's treatment programs may have referrals to therapists who are experienced at working with trauma survivors and careful about maintaining boundaries.

During ongoing recovery, you have the opportunity to look at past experiences that stand in the way of your own awakening and expansion. Although it takes a great deal of courage to face and tend to the pain without relying on the substances or behaviors that have numbed it, it is always worth the effort.

Your Sexual Rights and Responsibilities

Survivors of sexual trauma often gravitate toward one of two extremes. They may become sexually isolated, withdrawn, and avoidant, or they may become sexually active in a self-destructive way.

CSA survivors experience adult forms of sexual contact at an early age, and many learn little about sexually appropriate behavior. While they are still very young, they may act out sexually with other children. Many CSA survivors report having felt uncertain as teenagers about the appropriate progression of sexual contact in dating, which resulted in a reputation for being sexually promiscuous. It is also common for women who were sexually abused as children to experience later abuse by another authority figure.

The experience of violation of our sexual boundaries can become a reason to start actively pushing past the sexual boundaries of others—this begins as a way to take back control. Unfortunately, rather than return us to equilibrium, out-of-control sexual behavior can result. Adult survivors of SA may find themselves expressing sexual feelings even when it may not be welcome or appropriate.

On the other hand, lack of sexual desire is also a common complaint of sexual trauma survivors, along with a variety of other problems related to arousal. Many women go numb at a certain point in experiencing sexual excitement, others disconnect or dissociate from their bodies and find themselves unable to feel, and some experience flashbacks or sudden images of an abusive situation. All these experiences interfere with sexual pleasure and may make sex anxiety-provoking and painful.

The physical sexual repercussions of sexual trauma are often serious. In addition to the potential for injury, survivors may struggle later with lubrication, orgasm, painful intercourse, and vaginal spasms or vaginismus. Survivors of all genders may find parts of their body feel numb or untouchable. These and other symptoms are the body's way of saying that sex is not safe. Your body's memories of sexual trauma may override your emotional desires, making it feel extremely difficult for you to engage in any kind of sex.

Sexual trauma survivors often learn to put the sexual needs of another ahead of their own. They learned that their own needs and feelings were not important, and that to secure the love of another, or safety from further violation, they had to endure sexual contact they didn't want. As adults, many survivors place primary importance on their partner's experience and remain out of touch with their own needs and desires.

It is not uncommon for sexual trauma survivors to identify their own pleasure with pleasing their partner. Even for those who remain deeply invested in their partner's pleasure, as in many power exchange or kink relationships, it is important to be able to balance our focus and learn to enjoy our own experience during sexual connection.

Sexual trauma survivors may have been conditioned by negative sexual experiences to associate sex with helplessness, disgust, pain, anger, loss of control, shame, guilt, and even hate and rage. Therefore, it is often extremely difficult for survivors to experience sexuality with a deep sense of freedom. Sexual safety may not feel possible, or safety itself may not feel sexual.

The sexual challenges that result from sexual trauma do not go away by themselves. However, healing can occur, and survivors can make positive changes in their sexualities. Survivors can move out of old, self-defeating patterns that reinforce unsatisfying sexual experiences and move into experiencing the kinds of sexual lives that they want. One activity to support this process is to identify a set of sexual rights and responsibilities.

Your Sexual Rights and Responsibilities

Your list of sexual rights and responsibilities are yours to create. We recommend writing two lists that can be held side by side.

Some of your rights might include the right to say yes, the right to say no, the right to feel safe, the right to safer sex, the right to experiment, the right to choose your sex partner or multiple partners, the right to talk about sex, and the right to have limits.

Your responsibilities might include making sure you are listening to your partner when they say yes and no, initiating conversations about safer sex and making decisions together, listening to your own body and not pushing yourself past what feels good to you, and communicating with your partner about your desires and fears related to sex.

Go through your list of sexual rights and note each one that is not now an integral part of your sexual life. Ask yourself why you don't feel you have that right. Explore why you might be afraid to have that right, or what other form of resistance you may have. Visualize yourself having that right and see what you would have to do to create it for yourself.

Do the same for the responsibilities. Are you afraid to step up to the conversations about sex you may need to have with a new or established partner? If so, see if you can find a way to create more safety for yourself in those conversations—more on this in chapter 11.

When Michelle created her list of rights and responsibilities, she was overwhelmed with guilt and fear. She realized how many times she had had sex with her husband, Chris, when she didn't want to, whether out of a sense of obligation or to avoid a conflict when she was drunk, and it was difficult for her to face. She thought of herself as the more sexual partner in their marriage, but during her sobriety, she realized she had often thought of sex as a way to keep him happy and distract him from her drinking. As a couple, they had not been focusing on her pleasure, and she wanted to talk with Chris about this without hurting his pride.

Because Michelle had been practicing self-compassion, she was able to remind herself that what she had done in the past was what she thought best in the moment, and now she was equipped to make new choices. She was still afraid that if she told her husband she wanted to do things differently, he would resist. He had been getting more of what he wanted overall, she thought, and she was concerned that he would be angry with her once they started talking about her right to say no.

She was surprised, then, when she brought up this issue in couple's therapy and he seemed relieved that they were finally going to talk about it. The therapist gently guided the conversation, and Michelle was able to express some dissatisfaction with their sexual habits. Even with many months of sobriety from alcohol, Michelle had felt this issue was too difficult to broach. Chris nodded along as she described their struggle to reconnect sexually after such a long time of avoiding each other.

"Sometimes I'm so relieved that he wants to have sex with me that I'll just go with it, even if I'm not physically turned on," Michelle said, and she felt the tears begin to rise. "I feel guilty. I feel stupid. I want better for me, for him, for us both. We used to just fall into bed with so much passion for each other."

Chris chimed in. "I never want to make you do something you don't really want to do. When I think about your assault, I feel disgusted by the man who hurt you, and I never, ever want to do anything that would hurt you." They were able to meet each other's gaze. This was something Michelle didn't know she needed to hear, but it was a huge relief and reassurance that her husband was thinking about her boundaries this way.

With time and care, Michelle and Chris started unpacking how fearful they both had been about their sexual connection. They both had experienced a sense of rejection, a fear of approaching their partner with desire, and a feeling of being stuck in old habits. Once they were able to speak these honest feelings out loud, they could begin to create new ways to communicate, support each other, and explore new ways to connect sexually.

Even if sexual trauma has powerfully affected your ability to experience sexual pleasure, the healing available to you is just as powerful. Reclaiming your sexuality from an abusive past is possible. You have the right to enjoy your unique sexuality.

Beyond Self-Punishment

Those of us in recovery often experience guilt and shame about events that were not under our control, like CSA and SA. We also feel guilt and shame about behaviors that we feel we chose or could have prevented. Many of our experiences in life will be a confusing mix of both factors we were in control of and factors we weren't. This can be especially difficult for us to process when they are sexual experiences.

Most people who experience CSA and SA will not see their abusers/attackers take any responsibility or endure real consequences. The very few who use the criminal legal system may face a series of painful, retraumatizing events as they come to recognize the harm that was caused. This lack of community accountability leaves many of us feeling unsettled, and often we turn our pain back inward. In the absence of justice, we are more likely to punish ourselves.

Self-punishment is not the same as coming to terms with the abuse we experienced. We must move away from constant self-punishment, even if we have not yet been forgiven for everything we were responsible for, even if we wish we could tell a story about the past in which we were in control at all times, knowing deep down that we simply weren't. No one is in control of everything that happens to them all the time.

The way we characterize our own behavior matters for our ongoing recovery. Taking responsibility for ourselves is different from relentless self-punishment. In the following two scenarios, consider how self-compassion makes it possible to move forward, even from the experience of intense guilt and shame.

Dwelling on the Past

After the initial work of becoming sober from mind-altering substances and building in regular practices to help maintain that sobriety, Nova started focusing on her sexuality. At first, she chose to abstain from sexual contact with partners so she could reconnect with her own body and desires. Quickly, she noticed that her sobriety from alcohol, cocaine, and amphetamines had opened the door for disordered eating, and she turned her focus to her relationship with food.

The first step toward change is always to stop living in constant shame, but sometimes we forget this. For Nova, the physically healthier she felt, the sadder and more ashamed she became of the sex she had had while drunk and high. She had never felt embarrassed or ashamed about her sexual body or sexual behavior before, but now she felt she had harmed herself, and she didn't know how to forgive herself for it. She didn't want to make anyone else feel ashamed of their own sexual choices, so she didn't share her feelings with anyone at first.

Nova looked at her past behavior and saw that she had engaged in sexual activities when she didn't want to, or when she didn't have true capacity to consent. She had done things while intoxicated that she wouldn't have done sober. She became obsessed with these incidents, internally punishing herself for them without realizing it.

While abstaining from sexual relationships, she began to see *all* her past sexual experiences in a negative light. She felt she had *never* been sexually authentic and had only been performing for others' enjoyment. She feared she had lost her own sexuality to the demands of the people she tried to please. She spoke unkindly to herself, thinking of herself as "reckless and stupid." She did not feel hopeful about recovering a sense of her own sexual desire.

The wake-up call came one day when Nova heard a few dancers chatting in the dressing room at the club where she worked.

"One of them was helping the other block a customer in her phone," Nova recalled. "It was so clear that blocking him was difficult not only because he had been a source of income, but because she had gotten emotionally attached. Her friend just kept reminding her that he had crossed a line, and a boundary was needed." It became clear to Nova that the "line" had been something sexual—she didn't pry but she could tell that the situation had been confusing, uncomfortable, and difficult. Something clicked, Nova said, about the intense weight of shame women can carry about sexuality, especially under the pressures of an adult entertainment job.

"I started telling myself that everything I did in the past, and everything that happened to me, was part of my story, and from then on, I got to make new choices about how I wanted to live. I forgave myself for putting myself in confusing and sometimes dangerous situations.

"I realized that I still loved the part of me that was fearless, adventurous, and eager to try new experiences." She told herself it was okay if she never wanted to have sex again. She told herself it was okay if she wanted to try being sexual with women. She told herself she was free to make new sexual choices at any time, and that she didn't need to fear getting lost in someone else, because her body was hers to care for and enjoy. Nova began to forgive herself and move on from self-punishment, recognizing that no matter what she chose to do next with her body, she would be able to take care of herself.

The "Bad" Mother

Mothers with substance use disorders are especially stigmatized by a society that places the welfare of children almost exclusively in the hands of women. Opening to pleasure and sexual connection can feel especially difficult for mothers who do not feel they deserve to make time and space for it.

In early recovery, the guilt parents experience about the parenting they did while actively drinking or using often causes them to deny that their behavior affected their parenting at all. We have heard women say, "My babies weren't affected by my drinking—they were too young to know," "I did everything a good mother does, and I never got high in front of them," and "My daughter came first; I took care of her the same as any parent would."

Children are inevitably affected by their parents' out-of-control behaviors, no matter how hard the parents may try to be "perfect" when they are aware the kids are watching.

In ongoing recovery, these same parents are equipped to honestly look at the effects of their parenting. Empowerment about parenting means moving out of guilt and shame and taking responsibility for what happened in the past, as well as what is happening now. Women who don't resolve their guilt and shame often overcompensate in recovery, striving to be perfect mothers.

There's only one problem: To be a perfect mother you must have perfect children. Your children will be under tremendous pressure to behave well and to have only positive feelings so that they will reflect well on your parenting. They won't be allowed to be human, to express their full range of feelings and behavior.

This is a no-win situation both for the parent and for the children. The children will always fail because, as human beings, they can never be perfect. The parent, who must also fail in the attempt to be perfect, continues along the downward spiral of guilt and failure.

During her recovery process, Michelle found herself stuck in this spiral. One of her children began having some troubling behaviors when he entered first grade, and she could not shake her suspicion that his struggle was a direct result of her problems with alcohol. "If I'd been more present when he was little, more able to help him understand what he was feeling or teach him better coping skills," she would say, "I don't think he would be acting out so much now."

To break out of this pattern, Michelle first needed to accept and forgive herself for the quality of her parenting while she was drinking. She struggled to accept that her past was not what she would now choose, but she also saw how her struggle to forgive herself kept her from moving forward, to become the kind of parent she wanted to be.

Many women raised in families with challenges like substance use disorders and trauma feel inadequate to the task of parenting the way they wish. For some, parenting classes or support from a therapist or social worker can be indispensable help. Michelle leaned heavily on her sponsor and her women's group for support and advice while she worked through her guilt and shame about her parenting. She and Chris began to talk more openly about their hopes and goals for their family, and how to balance everyone's needs and desires with what was best for the whole.

Chris often reminded Michelle that a good mother is also one who takes care of herself. She was able to focus on her recovery, including getting exercise, eating well, getting enough sleep, spending time alone, and taking time for sober outings with her friends, in part because he was a dedicated and involved father.

For those of us who do not have partners, building a network of care is even more important. Single parenting is fundamentally stressful for most people, and creating a community of reliable, responsible people who can share the load should be a priority for parents in recovery.

Perhaps like Michelle, you can join a group that is a safe place to discuss how the issues of recovery and parenting come together, a place where you can express your concerns and feelings about your parenting responsibilities.

Being a responsible parent also means taking some responsibility for your children's recovery process. If they are grown, this may not be realistic. But if they still live with you at home, you can consider providing them with age-appropriate information about substance use issues or trauma and how it has affected you and the family.

Children may need to be in a counseling group or take part in individual or family therapy. Strange as it may seem, children can have a tough time adjusting to a parent's sobriety, and they may resent your attempts to resume the parental role. They may be very angry at what they perceive as their parent's prior neglect and abandonment, and they may need a safe place to work through these feelings.

After you have been in recovery for a while, you may discover that one or more of your children has been a victim of CSA. A very high percentage of sexually abused children come from families with substance use challenges, and it is extremely important that you not be in denial about that possibility with your children.

If you discover evidence of sexual abuse of your children, you must identify the abuser and make certain that they no longer have access to your children. This may be especially difficult if the abuser is a family member; but it is absolutely essential that your children know that you will protect them and that you will put their needs first. Although you were incapable of protecting them in the past, you can protect them now. You need to take an active stand on their behalf so you can start a healing process together.

Ongoing recovery is a time of deeper changes. As the layers of guilt and shame begin to peel away, and you develop more self-compassion, you can connect more with your current desires. Your capacity to know how you feel is directly related to your ability to consciously experience your body's sensations. When you are engaged with your body's sensations, you are listening to how your body responds to both your external and internal environments. Tuning in to your sensations without judgment is part of cultivating compassion for yourself.

You can create a sense of personal sexual dignity, empowering yourself to act on your sexuality without violating or coercing others, and becoming accountable for your sexual self and your recovery. Working with the issues that have kept you from empowerment and responsibility, such as shame, will enable you to experience intimacy with yourself and with those you love. As you grow in self-compassion, your capacity for pleasure will also grow.

◦ ◦ ◦

PART

4

Awakening to Intimacy

Experiencing authentic intimacy is one of the most hope-filled and exhilarating aspects of being human. As we progress in our healing, we are more able to experience the kind of trust between individuals that produces equality, mutuality, and reciprocity. Intimacy is a form of connection that deepens and enriches our lives. It is something we can feel with ourselves and in relationships with others. Developing these dynamics between yourself and others is a lifelong task.

Awakening to intimacy and awakening to your sexuality are interrelated. Both are dimensions of the ongoing process of recovery. In recovery we begin to understand what we have longed for, what we really want in our lives. This next level of awakening poses an exciting challenge for all of us, no matter where we are on this path.

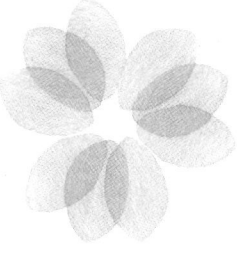

CHAPTER 10

Developing Self-Intimacy

Be willing to look in every corner and under
all the rugs and closets to find the lost parts
of you that were stashed and swept into
the cracks and crannies. They are waiting
for the thick medicinal salve of your patient,
loving attention. Stay with your heart
in all weather. Stay warm.

———

Pixie Lighthorse, *The Wound Makes the Medicine:
Elemental Remediations for Transforming Heartache*

What is intimacy? A simple way to think of it is deep, honest, safe, trusting connection that brings a sense of joy and satisfaction to our lives. As we move toward establishing real intimacy in our relationships, it becomes clear that intimacy with ourselves is our foundation for intimacy with others.

Our quest for healthier forms of self-care and self-love can feel exhausting and never-ending, in part because these ideals have been co-opted by market forces that profit from our attempts. While we may benefit from investment in therapy, recovery programs, books, classes, gym memberships, and other forms of self-care, ultimately self-intimacy is something we must discover within ourselves.

Most of us have so little real experience of intimacy that the word itself is baffling or surrounded by fear and mistrust. Sometimes we use it as a euphemism for sex. We say, "I'm having an intimate relationship with someone," which society understands as, "We're having sex." But it's not the same thing. Not even close.

Like sexuality, intimacy is complex. There are different ways of experiencing and expressing it. Emotional intimacy involves sharing our feelings; intellectual intimacy involves sharing our thoughts; physical intimacy involves sharing our bodies, not always in sexual ways.

We live in a society that confuses and mixes together love, sex, and intimacy. Often when we're looking for one, we go out and get another. When you're looking for intimacy, you may end up in a sexual encounter, but the fact that it is sexual does not make it intimate. Conversely, you may be very intimate with someone with whom you are not sexual at all.

Love is also a huge word, encompassing multiple forms of relationship: familial, romantic, friendship, and so on. We can feel love for someone without experiencing intimacy with them. Partnerships can be fluid too, sometimes filled with sexual connection and at other times not, while the love and intimacy remain. One partner may feel just as intimate without sexual connection, while the other requires sex to feel close. And on and on. This is why knowing yourself, being in tune with your own feelings, needs, and desires, and developing an intimate relationship with yourself is such an important part of recovery.

People in recovery from addictions and out-of-control behaviors must also contend with the damaging effects of the addictive process. Addiction prevents intimacy; it can destroy even the possibility of intimacy. An addictive relationship with anything or anyone is a relationship that is out of balance. The object of addiction—alcohol, drugs, food restriction, a person, spending, and so many others—becomes the focal point of life. In essence, it becomes the only thing one trusts and cares about. Even if the love object is a human being, as with imbalanced relationships or out-of-control sexual behavior, the objectification of that person renders intimacy impossible.

Addiction interferes with the ability to experience deep connection with others. Our perceptions become distorted, our behavior becomes defensive, our feelings become altered. In recovery we learn to recognize these processes in their early stages and change our direction. To know ourselves this deeply means taking responsibility for not only our behavior, but the thinking and feeling that leads us to it.

Being intimate with yourself does not mean being narcissistic, obsessing endlessly about yourself and your own wants and needs. It does not mean you have to focus on yourself to the exclusion of others. It means knowing who you are, being in touch with your feelings as they occur, and feeling curious about why you react to events and situations as you do. It means committing to your own sexual life, regardless of whether you are sharing physical connection with another person. It can mean sex with yourself, exploring your fantasies, and learning about what makes you excited. Self-intimacy is the practice of being your own best friend, partner, lover, and wise guide.

Knowing yourself includes knowing your feelings, body, mind, spirit, and sexuality. Ultimately, these are not discrete layers of you—they are all connected, overlapping and intertwined. As you move up the spiral of recovery and healing, you will discover more about who you are now, and who you are becoming.

Know Your Feelings

Feelings are inevitable. They are a valuable source of information about who we are and what we are experiencing. You do not have to judge them, deny them, or act upon them; it is enough to feel and observe them. You can decide how to take action after first spending time with your feelings.

In the wake of trauma or while caught up in addiction, people are generally accustomed to acting out their feelings without really being aware of them, and that acting out often has a compulsive quality. But as you allow yourself simply to feel your feelings, whether of sadness, anger, joy, or loss, you will lessen the need to act impulsively from them. Simply being with your feelings, noting them, and allowing them to exist within you can free you to be able to choose how to express them.

You may have compressed your feelings into one dominant feeling state. The most common after addiction and trauma are anger, hurt, fear, anxiety, shame, and numbness. This state may have become your constant way of being. You may have lost your ability to feel a wide range of feelings or to discriminate between feelings.

Ask yourself what dominant feeling you are experiencing. Are you angry or hurt? Disappointed, maybe frustrated? Fearful? If you are experiencing a more complex set of feelings, keep naming them. Some of your feelings might include irritation, delight, distress, abhorrence, heartache, satisfaction, dread, intolerance, excitement, and so on. Yes, there are likely a few positive feelings mixed in.

While many people prefer to think of feelings as either good or bad, there are hundreds of words that describe the many different feelings, shades of feelings, nuances of feelings. Some feelings are complex all on their own, like nostalgia, which is a bittersweet experience of affection for a time in the past. Sometimes we have multiple feelings at once, all asking for attention and expression. When a baby is born, for example, a heady mix of joy, awe, anxiety, and sometimes grief for the way life used to be can all be present at the same time.

Countless lists of feelings are available online, including some that are color-coded and quite nuanced. If you are having trouble identifying your feelings, this is a good place to start. You can search for "feelings wheel," "wheel of emotions," or "list of feelings" and see what makes the most sense to you.

It is not possible to control our feelings so thoroughly that we avoid the ones we experience as "bad" or uncomfortable. Feelings do not operate like a faucet—we can't turn on the warm side and leave the cold side off. When we are ready to thaw out and feel our feelings, we are going to feel both the pleasant and unpleasant. With time, practice, and care, even uncomfortable feelings become an opportunity for self-knowledge and self-intimacy. As we gain self-supportive skills and tolerance for our intense feelings, we become more able to connect with our own lives and other people.

Many recovering people have a lifetime of stored-up, unexpressed feelings buried underneath today's mood. It is common to repress big feelings like grief or rage, because we fear being overwhelmed and engulfed by their intensity and strength. Many of our families offered both direct and indirect messages that told us not to identify and express feelings. Luckily, the skills of identifying, experiencing, and choosing how to express feelings can be developed at any time.

In recovery, access to feelings can be more immediate. Without the dampening-down effect of addiction or compulsive behavior, unexpressed feelings may come rushing to the surface. If you become easily overwhelmed, you may need to choose a guide, like a therapist, or another safe container, like a process group, to help you grow in tolerance of the uncomfortable feelings. Like waves, feelings will ebb and flow. In time, feelings can be less fearsome, and they can teach us about ourselves. New feelings can be welcomed into our lives as precious life experience.

There is great value in being connected to old feelings in order to dissipate them. When you allow old feelings to dissolve, what you feel in the present moment is about what is happening today. While reading this book and engaging with the exercises, you have likely begun to clear out some older feelings. Making space for new emotional experiences is a key part of awakening your sexuality.

Know Your Body

When you are disconnected and estranged from your body, you are missing a valuable source of self-knowledge and self-understanding. Your body is a treasury of knowledge about yourself. How and what your body feels can tell you a great deal about what's going on with you. Often, feelings you don't express emotionally find expression through your body. Headaches, stomachaches, backaches, muscle tension, hypertension, and breathing disorders may all be signals that a strong feeling needs your attention.

Because we most often express our sexuality with our body, knowing our body precedes a full knowledge of who we are as expressive sexual beings. In previous chapters, you learned the importance of accepting your body. Through the practice of self-intimacy, awareness gradually develops of your own sexual responses as separate from a partner's. In ongoing recovery, you begin to assert your body's needs in relation to the needs of others.

Now you can build on your knowledge of your own body and its responses and begin to explore some areas of your sexuality that may have lain dormant. You may enjoy nonsexual activities, such as dancing or walking outdoors, that make your body feel good. You may expand your ability to touch others and yourself with a greater variety of techniques and approaches, and you may become more flexible in your sexual responses and behaviors.

The idea that the body and emotions are intimately connected is not a new one, but today we are even more aware of the subtle interaction between the two. Whether you are feeling happy, sad, fearful, vibrant, exhausted, frustrated, angry, or forgiving, your body contains the feeling. Your unexpressed feelings are your body's burden to bear. One way to think about feelings is that they must be metabolized, like food. What is nutritive will be used, and what is not nourishing needs to be passed through the body. We exhale, cry, laugh, shake, sleep, sweat, and excrete—feelings can affect and be affected by all these processes.

Paying loving attention to our body is an important avenue to identifying our feelings. Often pain is the only way our body can tell us that something is wrong. Rather than pushing through pain and ignoring the signs that our body is offering us, sexual recovery asks us to slow down and listen, and give our body what it needs. While breath, food, water, and shelter are first-order human needs to stay alive, we have other needs that also must be met for us to thrive. These include movement, connective touch, and time spent in natural space.

Movement

Energetic, joyful physical activity, such as dance, or slow, thoughtful physical activity, such as yoga, can release emotions in surprising ways. One woman told us, "Every time I would do a particular yoga pose, I would feel very, very sad and begin to cry. To this day, I don't know why that pose brought on that response, but it did serve to release that sadness and bring it to my attention so I could work on it."

Patterned, rhythmic, repetitive movement is key to processing emotions. The movement that works for you will be unique to your body. One of the most accessible, to most people, is walking. Even a short ten-minute walk can help bring you back to yourself. You can also bounce a ball against a wall, sway your body side to side, or pat your body gently from head to toe. If you enjoy more intense physical sensations, you can lift weights, try a martial art, or attend a group fitness class. Engaging in a movement practice is not about getting exercise, although that can be a benefit. It is about movement, period. Moving the body encourages movement of feelings.

Connective Touch

For those who are engaging in sexual recovery while maintaining partnerships, touch may be a place where the partner can be asked to participate. However, connective touch does not need to happen only in romantic and sexual partnerships. Recent research suggests that a lack of regular, daily connective touch has significant negative emotional and psychological impacts. If you do not have people near you whom you feel safe hugging, cuddling with, holding, or even sitting next to, it is time to seek them out.

If it is financially possible, seeking massage, acupressure, or other bodywork techniques may also help. There are communities in most cities dedicated to safe cuddling, where you can attend gatherings in which people practice consent, maintain boundaries, and offer each other supportive touch. Sometimes we think we need or want sex when it is connective touch we are seeking.

Co-author Vanessa has worked for more than twenty-five years in various adult industries, including in-person sex work. They recall a client who had a very busy life, a high-powered job, and many people who surrounded him daily. He did not seem starved for contact with people, but there were no intimate relationships in his life. "I always felt like the most important part of our time together was the ten minutes or so when I would hold him after sex," Vanessa remembers. "So one time I thought I'd try something different. I encouraged him to lie on his belly, and after massaging him for a short while, I lay on top of him, covering as much of his body as I could with my own. I put my full weight on him, rested my head on his upper back, arms on his arms, legs on his legs. He fell into a deep sleep almost immediately. When he woke up a few minutes later, he was astonished. He told me he had no idea how badly he'd needed that."

We can't always perceive our own need for touch the way we feel our need for food and water, but it is a need. The language we use reveals this: "skin hunger" and "touch starvation" are the two most common ways to describe a person who is lacking in regular connective touch.

While many people are touch-starved, some are touched-out. For parents of small children, partners of people who ask for constant physical contact, and those for whom touch is simply not preferable, it can be difficult to initiate touch without feeling depleted. Importantly, connective touch is replenishing and nourishing for you—it does not require you to expend significant energy. Sometimes connective touch is mutual, and sometimes you receive it via a professional or the focused attention of a person who cares for you. It does not need to be sustained for long periods of time to be helpful—even one truly supportive hug makes a big difference. Part of self-intimacy is identifying your own needs for touch. Are you in need of more connective, supportive touch from other people? Do you know how to offer it to yourself?

When you do not have the option of connective touch with another person, you can give yourself some of the touch you need. Begin with a self-hug, wrapping yourself in your own arms and holding yourself firmly. Take three full breaths in and out before you release.

Time in Nature

Your body is not separate from the natural world; it is part of it. Some people have consistent contact with the natural space around them—they live or work in places where plants, animals, soil, sky, and seasons are part of everyday life. Increasingly, more humans live in cities, where regular contact with nature is more difficult to come by. In most cities, there is some green space afforded to the public in the way of parks, trails, walkways, or playgrounds. You don't need a large expanse of mind-blowing mountains; you just need to regularly prioritize putting your body closer to the natural world. You can stop and watch an ant as it makes its way across a bench. You can slip your shoes off and put your feet in the grass. You can sniff the scent of the earth after a rain. Look up into the sky at night and notice the moon.

As part of her recovery process from sexual trauma, one woman told us she "got seriously into" herbalism. A set of herbal remedies recommended by an herbalist in her town had helped her with her insomnia, lack of appetite, and muscle aches while she withdrew from alcohol. She became curious about how plants have been used for thousands of years by humans everywhere to remedy common ailments, and she got excited to study the art of botanical medicine that was part of her own heritage. "My grandmother never taught me what she knew," she told us. "But I found a 'curandera' from a similar region in Mexico, and I'm hearing her say the names of plants I haven't heard since I was a little girl. I feel like I'm involved in something old and sacred, and also, it's just fun! Every time I go out for a walk, I am saying hello to the plants the way I would say hello to old friends."

Know Your Mind

Becoming familiar with your thinking can be very exciting, and it can also bring awareness of difficult inner dialogue. As you tune into your body, you will likely also be hearing from your mind. Ongoing recovery invites you to investigate how your mind works, what triggers a thought process, how you solve problems, what prevents you from thinking clearly about an issue, and more. Exploring your intellectual capacities may be a new experience. Or perhaps like Tamara, who earned a PhD and became a professor, the world of the mind is your safe refuge. Wherever your experience falls, getting to know your own mind is an important feature of your self-intimacy.

Alcohol and most mood-altering substances can make it very difficult to think clearly. If you are recovering from addiction, you will likely find yourself thinking more clearly as you reduce or stop your use. As your recovery progresses, you may find that you are more able to concentrate, you are less forgetful, and you are more present to your own thoughts.

Trauma also alters our thinking. Many trauma survivors are unaware of how negatively they speak to themselves internally. Speaking kindly to yourself in your mind may be a new or uncomfortable experience, but the practice is invaluable.

Recovering your thinking self can be one of the most satisfying experiences of recovery. You may find yourself taking on new intellectual challenges, going back to school, or learning new skills as a result of honoring your mind and its capabilities. You are reading this book and processing the information—that is an important accomplishment!

Understanding your mind's abilities and awareness of how your mind works are part of your path to greater self-intimacy. Remember that self-compassion needs to lead the way. You get to decide which of your thoughts best indicates who you are, and you do not need to overidentify with self-harming or unwanted thoughts. If you find that your mind is constantly criticizing you or others, flashing ahead to scary future possibilities, or stuck replaying painful past events, you may need to recruit more support. Anxiety, depression, and symptoms like intrusive thoughts can overwhelm the mind. If the thoughts feel too powerful and lead to overwhelming feelings, it is time to ask for help.

As you reclaim your thinking, you will also begin to clarify your thoughts on sex. You may begin to see how your sexual thinking affects your choices. You may observe when you lapse into imagining the future and making assumptions about possible sexual interactions.

One night Michelle told her group, "Last night, I really felt like having sex. But I said to myself, 'I'm sure Chris isn't feeling it, so why bother?' And then suddenly I realized that this entire situation was inside my own head. I had no idea what Chris was feeling." Like Michelle, in ongoing recovery, you will become more and more aware of your sexual thoughts and assumptions and how they affect your actions.

This ability to notice our own thoughts is a foundational aspect of mindfulness. You have already practiced tuning into your body's sensations, which is another mindfulness practice. In her book *Better Sex Through Mindfulness: How Women Can Cultivate Desire*, Dr. Lori Brotto writes that "all of the skills practiced in mindful awareness—noticing bodily sensations, being aware of the breath, observing sounds and thoughts—can be directly applied to sexual activity."[1] Brotto's research shows that mindfulness practices can improve women's experience of sexual desire and pleasure, and even reduce the experience of pain with sex, reduce anxiety about low sexual desire, and improve overall well-being. Your efforts to become more aware of your body and mind are directly linked to your capacity to enjoy sexual feelings.

As a woman recovering from opioid addiction and still living with chronic pain, Tamara was motivated to seek out new methods for managing her body's discomfort. Her insurance covered a pain specialist who helped her transition to non-opioid pain medications, and that doctor recommended she look into mindfulness meditation as a supplemental support.

Tamara took her powerful intellect to the task, researching the effectiveness of mindfulness meditation and reading books and articles written by practitioners and neuroscientists. She had already attended a lecture at her university on the current neuroscience of addiction, and she was able to reach out to a researcher in the psychology department for recommendations about research into mindfulness meditation and chronic pain.

When Tamara discovered that mindfulness had been shown to significantly reduce chronic pain in both experimental and clinical settings, she was amazed. Tamara began a practice under the tutelage of a local mindfulness meditation practitioner. Adding this piece to her recovery repertoire opened the door for a new level of self-awareness and joy in her own life. Tamara still dealt with her chronic pain and disability from her car accident, but she began to feel more alive in her body and senses, more connected to how her mind worked, and more interested in what her life might bring next. One specific gift of her practice was the way it helped her relearn how to breathe deeply and slowly.

The mind is not separate from the body. Bodily processes affect how we think, and breathing is a process that has direct and immediate effects. You may discover that you have been holding your breath without realizing it. This can manifest as hyperventilating, faintness, chest pains, and headaches. You may be doing this in response to anxieties rooted in either the past or the future. As you learn to live in the present, you will become aware of your breath patterns. If you are feeling anxious or depressed, taking time out to breathe quietly and slowly is a good way to bring yourself back to the present.

Staying in the present takes practice and attention, but it is rewarding. The more you try to do it, the more you will be able to do it. At first you may be able to be present only for a second or two, then a minute or two. Soon you will begin to notice when you have been lost in a dream of the past or future, and you will be able to gently return yourself to the present, to what is actually happening right here, right now. This is the dawning of a new self-awareness.

Know Your Spirit

A fundamental part of knowing yourself is knowing your spiritual self, investigating that part of who you are that connects you to something larger. Whether you think of this mysterious aspect as God or Goddess, Higher Power, consciousness, electrical impulses in the brain, a reincarnated soul, the connectedness of life on Earth, or something else—that is something you decide for yourself. We use the term *spirit* here because it captures an idea, but of course that idea may not fit in with your beliefs. If *spirit* doesn't sound right for you, please feel free to imagine simply the facts: Each of us is always part of something larger than ourselves, and we are alive now because of the generations of people who lived before us.

People find their way to a sense of interconnectedness in infinite ways. You may find yours in nature, in meditation, or in prayer. You may set time aside for devotional reading or silence. You may try psychedelic medicine therapy with an experienced guide, or you may practice savoring your coffee in the morning. Whatever form your practice takes, we encourage you to take the time to find those moments when you can feel the vitality of life in and around you.

It can be difficult to respect your spiritual needs in a society that appears so focused on the material, external, and urgent. Knowing yourself spiritually is not simply knowing what you believe; it also includes recognizing and validating your longings by taking time out of your busy life to fulfill those needs. As you search for wholeness, harmony, and connection to yourself, other people, and the world, you will come to know who you are. You will develop a deeper understanding of what it means to you to be alive in this body for the time that you have.

The feeling of ecstasy, which we tend to connect with physical pleasure, was considered by many ancients to be a merging with the divine, truly heaven on earth. In ongoing recovery, you will learn to honor the sexual part of yourself as an irreplaceable and integral aspect of the sacredness of your being.

Know Your Sexuality

For some people, sexual identity is clear and fixed—they have certainty about whom they are attracted to and what they do and do not enjoy, and they can name the reasons why they might want to have sex. For many others, sexual identity is not quite so predictable and defined. If you are still learning about your sexual self, take heart. As time passes and your needs change, your sexual identity will reflect this change.

Knowing your sexuality does not mean defining yourself with a label and never revising it. Knowing your sexuality means giving awareness and attention to your feelings, allowing yourself to have fantasies and desires that surprise you, and listening to what your body tells you. You may experience change in the kinds of sexual behavior you enjoy and the types of people you are attracted to, including becoming attracted to another gender.

Although our society socializes us to be exclusively heterosexual for our whole lives, the reality of human sexual identity is a complex and varied spectrum. You are free to explore your sexual identity without having to categorize yourself into a rigid definition that may not fit your experience or feelings. At the same time, for some people, having labels feels important and safe—it validates their experience and helps them feel connected to a community.

Sex researchers have tried various ways to help people define and describe their sexuality, including the Kinsey Scale for sexual identity, the Klein Sexual Orientation Grid, and the Sell Assessment of Sexual Orientation. As more people speak up about their complex experience of sexuality and gender, the more terms, labels, and possibilities we create. However you identify—straight, gay, lesbian, bisexual, queer, pansexual, asexual, or any other orientation, you deserve to use the terms that feel right for you.

Sexual orientation—whom you are attracted to—is only one facet of your sexual identity. For many, sexual attraction and romantic attraction are linked, as in, the people they are attracted to sexually are the same people they would want to be in a romantic relationship with. However, this is not the case for everyone. Some people find that their sexual attractions are distinct from their romantic or relational attractions. Some people are polyamorous or nonmonogamous as part of their identity, and others may enter nonmonogamous relationships without adopting an identity label. Many people have partnerships that are emotionally intimate with only one person but allow sexual nonmonogamy as part of the relationship. Some deeply identify with kink or BDSM and find satisfaction either sexually or relationally (or both) in forms of sexual play that fall outside societal norms. Truly, the possibilities are endless.

Sexuality is also distinct from gender. Your understanding of your gender may change with time and experience. Maybe you have always known your gender and have been comfortable with it, or maybe you haven't expressed it fully. For Ash, coming out as nonbinary was both freeing and difficult. They felt as though they were bringing a more honest and full version of themself to the world, but because so many people they knew struggled to understand what "nonbinary" gender meant, or to use they/them pronouns easily, it was difficult to decide how to navigate the constant misunderstandings, misgendering, and questions that came up. The world around Ash was built for a gender binary: men, women, and that's it. This made Ash feel as though their true self was not valid or wanted, except in queer community space where nonbinary people could gather more safely.

While sexuality and gender are distinct, they do not exist wholly independently. Questions about gender can be intertwined with our sexuality too. One trans woman told us that her attraction to women made her gender identity more difficult for her to understand as a younger person. "Kids teased me about being gay," she said, "but I wasn't a gay boy. I was a girl who liked girls, who still was living my life as a boy. It was too much for most people I knew to even understand, including myself, for a long time."

No one really knows how any particular sexual identity develops. The only facts we're clear about are that all sexual identities are valid, that they can be complex, and that they can change and develop over time. Whether you feel sure or uncertain, new to this conversation or experienced, spending some time asking yourself the following questions is a valuable exercise in knowing your sexuality more deeply.

My Sexuality: Past, Present, and Future

You may want to answer these questions three times: once for the version of you in the past who was not involved in a recovery process, once for who you are today, and once for your ideal future—where you'd like to be. These three sets of answers will give you some idea of how your sexual identity has developed and the direction you'd like to move in. Start with where you are today.

- **Fantasies:** Who and what are your fantasies about? Do you fantasize about particular acts with particular people? If you do not currently fantasize, did you do so in the past? Can you remember when or why you stopped? If you never have, what does it feel like to try? Are there any books, movies, shows, music, or other media that fuel your fantasies?

- **Eroticism:** What feels erotic to you? Are there particular bodies you find more erotic than others? Do you find particular physical characteristics erotic? Can you feel erotic with yourself alone? Do you feel erotic when out in nature, dancing, eating a rich meal, or . . . ? Do you feel excited by feelings of danger, humiliation, degradation, dominance, or control? Are there particular smells, tastes, textures, or sounds that are erotic for you?

- **Emotional attachments:** Where do your strongest emotional attachments lie? Are you equally attached to people of different genders, or do you find your strongest attachments tend to be with a certain gender? Whom are your emotional bonds and connections with? Whom do you wish to connect with?

- **Sexual behavior:** What is your sexual experience? With whom have you had sexual activity? Does your sexual experience align with what you find erotic? Are there sexual experiences you want to have for the first time or repeat from the past? What are your habits and patterns around masturbation?

Now answer the questions again. This time, try to recreate your experiences prior to entering recovery, and see how your sexual identity has shifted with recovery. Then answer the questions again with an eye toward the future. What would you like to explore? How would you like to develop sexually?

It can be difficult to face the impacts of sexual trauma on our capacity for pleasure, desire, intimacy, and connection. There may have been a time in the past when you felt more curious, free, and safe with sex. Or there may have been very few times in which you felt innocent, especially if you experienced CSA. Answering these questions can reveal places where your sexual self has been stuck, hiding, or afraid. Remember that self-knowledge does not need to be put into practice immediately. You can stay gentle with yourself and make changes that feel safe.

When Nova did this exercise, she was surprised to realize that she mostly had fantasies about women, while the majority of her sexual experience was with men. Her main emotional attachments were also mostly with queer women and nonbinary people. She decided in the future to pay more attention to her sexual desires and to be more open to new erotic experiences and honor her emotional connections.

This exercise can also alert you to areas of sexuality where you are curious but need more education. Finding good information about sexuality can feel overwhelming. You can begin with the list of resources at the end of this book and see where your explorations take you.

Conscious Masturbation

Knowing your sexuality and knowing what your body looks and feels like during sexual arousal go hand in hand. In chapter 4, you took a look at your genitals in the mirror. Now, you can explore your body's sexual responses with even more gentle curiosity.

Begin by setting yourself up well: Get as physically comfortable as you can, in a time and place when you are able to have privacy. Set up a mirror so you can watch how your genitals change with arousal. We highly recommend using a lubricant—any type that works for your body. If you have physical limitations that prevent you from reaching your genitals with your hands, please use any assistive devices you may already have. If you are used to masturbating with a vibrator, feel free to have it handy.

Begin with soft, gentle strokes, and move slowly. For a vulva, move from outer labia to inner. Notice if your skin color changes with arousal; notice any changes with increased blood flow to your genitals. You may notice an increase in lubrication. Many women will be able to see when their clitoris enlarges and becomes erect, then later retracts and becomes hidden. For others, the visible change is not as pronounced, but the sensations usually change as the clitoris fills with blood.

When Tamara began this exercise, she thought it would be easy. She had been masturbating with orgasms—multiples, even—for many years, and she knew how to stimulate herself. But as she began to touch herself with the awareness required by this exercise, she was surprised to find that there were many aspects of giving herself pleasure that she had been ignoring.

She had always concentrated on getting to the orgasmic release as quickly as possible. Because of her back pain, she often held her body very rigidly during orgasm, afraid of hurting herself. Now Tamara began to enjoy the sensuality of her skin, touching and stroking her breasts, her stomach, her hips, teasing her own body as she might that of a lover. At the same time, she discovered that areas other than the head of her clitoris were also sensitive, and she gave attention to these as well. She gently massaged the rim of her vaginal opening, brushing her hand lightly over her pubic hair.

After several months, she grew to know her responses in a way that amazed her. She felt a deep sense of compassion and gratitude for how her body still felt pleasure, despite what she had been through.

Unlike Tamara, who came to this exercise with self-awareness and experience, Miyu had never had an orgasm. She had only recently learned that she could have any pleasurable sensation about herself connected with her body, much less one from her genitals. While Miyu had been able to recover from anorexia and self-harming, she had not found a way to open up her body to sexual pleasure.

When Miyu's sex education teacher informed her that masturbation is the best way for preorgasmic women to learn how to have an orgasm, she was frightened. She had learned to look at her body in the mirror, and even to accept what she saw. She had learned to look at and even touch her genitals. But those seemed like clinical exercises. This was much more threatening. She was beginning to feel uncomfortable about the time she was spending with her own body.

Like Miyu, you may need to deal with feelings of repulsion about masturbation before you are able to move toward a more satisfying sexuality that includes orgasm. You may need to work through old feelings of guilt and shame. If, like Tamara, you have felt connected to your sexual body in the past, and aren't troubled by the idea of masturbation, then slowing down your exploration and experimenting with new sensations may open up deeper levels of connection to your sexuality in the present.

Trauma, compulsive behaviors, substance dependence, and the stress of beginning recovery all affect how our bodies respond to stimuli, even our familiar ways of masturbating. For example, one woman who did this exercise realized that she had been masturbating with a very strong vibrator for years, thinking that she had difficulty orgasming because her clitoris was "not that sensitive." It turned out that when she gave herself time to slowly become more aroused, and touched more of her own body with her hands, she wanted much less direct clitoral stimulation than she expected. She had developed her masturbation habits while using cocaine, and years later, her body had different needs. When she slowed down and allowed her body time to warm up, she had powerful orgasms with a less intense vibrator.

Knowing how to reliably bring yourself to orgasm means you can take responsibility for your own pleasure. When your partners no longer have to guess at what you're in the mood for and are relieved of the full responsibility of satisfying you sexually, they too are freed up to be more experimental and more responsive.

When you know what excites you and what brings you to orgasm, you can begin to communicate this clearly to your partners.

Self-intimacy is rooted in self-knowledge. Knowing your own body, mind, spirit, and sexuality, especially when you can view what you find through the lens of self-compassion, creates space for sexual flourishing. You may choose to continue this journey on your own, or from inside a preexisting partnership. You will be entering a new phase of your life in which you build your relationships on a stronger foundation. The next chapter will focus on how you can bring your new skills into relationships with other people.

○ ○ ○

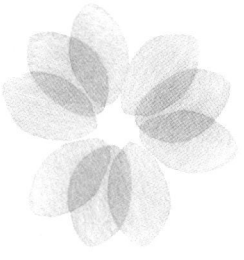

CHAPTER 11

Creating Deeper
Connections with Others

*If we were constantly remembering that love
is as love does, we would not use the word
in a manner that devalues and degrades its
meaning. When we are loving, we openly and
honestly express care, affection, responsibility,
respect, commitment, and trust.*

———

bell hooks, *All About Love: New Visions*

G reat sex can happen in a wide variety of circumstances— with or without intimacy, with someone you barely know or know extremely well, spontaneously or after careful planning. However, a great sexual *relationship* is nourishing, sustaining, pleasurable, and growth-fostering. It takes skill to maintain. The first skill is friendship.

For those who are currently partnered, this chapter will offer tools for creating greater intimacy in current relationships. For those seeking new romantic and sexual relationships, this chapter will lay the groundwork for creating honest connections that can flourish over time, with care. For those who are not seeking sexual partnership at this time, this chapter will affirm the importance of cultivating intimacy in friendships.

Getting to know your unique sexuality in the present is the most important action you can take in the journey toward intimacy with others. If during your explorations so far you have determined that you want to refrain from sharing your sexual self with a partner for any reason, this chapter can still apply to your life. As it turns out, building multiple forms of meaningful connections, such as the love we feel with friends, can be key to sexual recovery, even for people who are on the asexuality spectrum or are abstaining from partner sex for any other reason.

Nourishing Friendships

Have you ever noticed a friend of yours who seems to disappear each time she is dating someone new? Or perhaps you are that person who finds it difficult to maintain your friendships when there is a new partner in your life. Many people find themselves concentrating on their sexual relationships to the detriment of their friendships.

Taking the time to nurture and maintain our friendships is not easy, but it is essential to our sustenance and nourishment. Having a friend who has known you and supported you over time, no matter how frequently or infrequently you see one another, helps to remind you of the reality of your experiences, the continuity of your life, and your value and presence in someone else's life. Maintaining friendships is also part of maintaining your independent self and can help prevent you from getting lost in someone new.

While some friendships may include sexual attraction and even be sexual relationships, this discussion is about friendships that do not include sexuality as a feature. At the same time, it is important to note that the qualities we develop and deepen in friendship are the same ones that can make our long-term sexual relationships meaningful: honesty, vulnerability, support, playfulness, curiosity, commitment, mutuality, and shared power.

Respect, Mutuality, and Compassion

There are as many ways to be friends as there are human beings. Some friendships may have inherent power differences, like mentorships, friendships with a significant age difference, friendships among people who have very different financial situations, or friendships formed within hierarchies at work.

When power is unequal, it is common for the one with less power to learn more about the other partner than vice versa. In our society, the poor know more about the middle class, who, in turn, study the rich; people of color know more about white people, women know more about men, transgender people know more about cisgender people, and so on. To be truly intimate, friends must be conscious of and tenderly work though the feelings that come up about the social inequalities and power differences that may exist among them.

The lack of social equality among men, women, and nonbinary and gender-expansive people can make friendship difficult. Yet many of us are striving to create deeply connective, nourishing friendships. This means navigating our differences with curiosity, compassion, and care.

In mutual relationships, we experience a reciprocal interest in giving and receiving. We each have a mutual desire to create and maintain the relationship. We both find the friendship important and value it in a similar manner. In a mutual friendship, we express similar degrees of vulnerability and ability to trust. We both put energy into being together and listening to and supporting each other. No wide disparity exists between how much each of us works to maintain the relationship.

In a close friendship, we act as mirrors for each other. If I see you doing something, I can ask myself without judgment, "Do I do that too? Is it what I want to be doing?" We become more empathic as we see ourselves mirrored in each other.

On the other hand, we also learn about ourselves from seeing the reactions our own behavior stimulates. An intimate friend can help you recognize when their response was not provoked by anything you did but was about something entirely different and separate from you. Also, the same friend might be able to help you understand how something you've said or done has had a negative impact. The mirroring of an intimate friendship allows us to know ourselves better.

In friendship, you can allow yourself to be seen and heard and to really see and hear another person. You can allow yourself to be influenced by and to influence someone else. You are willing to both act upon and be acted upon. You can share your inner thoughts, feelings, desires, and needs with those you are close to. Thus your inner and outer lives meet and become whole, which is an essential experience to your recovery.

The rewards of friendships that endure over time are great. Our friends see us change and grow, and they can provide us with an understanding that comes only with years of connection. Abiding friends have been with us through numerous ups and downs, like family struggles, job changes, illnesses, accomplishments. They can provide us with continuity of intimacy in a time when sexual relationships may be difficult to sustain.

Within any particular friendship, there will be an ebb and flow to the pattern of closeness, times in both your lives in which you're closer and times you're more remote. Nonetheless, staying connected to friends over distance and time can provide you with strong and enduring bonds that can sustain you through the most difficult trials.

Some dear friendships cannot endure the changes that recovery brings. If your close friends are experiencing their own addiction or unaddressed trauma symptoms, your recovery may disrupt the status quo. You may need to make difficult choices about the time and effort you spend with friends who cannot support your recovery process or who were your companions for addictive behavior. Remember that as you have changed, so can others, and even if you need to create boundaries in the present, you can always reconsider them if your friend enters a recovery process of their own.

The emotional skills like boundaries, conflict resolution, and honest communication that you build in your friendships are also what will sustain your romantic and sexual relationships.

Dating New People

Talking about sexuality in early dating relationships can feel overwhelming, so much so that many people simply do not do it. If you are dating while sober, you may find that you used to rely on alcohol or other substances to bridge the gap between a flirtation and a sexual experience. Now you have to do it yourself, and it can be difficult to know where to start.

Those who use dating apps are navigating a sometimes bewildering set of questions when they start talking to someone new. While dating apps have made it more common for people to openly discuss their likes, dislikes, and relationship goals, they have not yet cured our culture of embarrassment, shame, and inequality when it comes to sexuality.

Large surveys show us that the pleasure gap is real. If we look at orgasms alone (only one way of measuring pleasure!), recent surveys indicate that 57 percent of women who have sex with men orgasm most or every time they have sex with a partner, while 95 percent said their male partner orgasms most or every time.[1] The difference in orgasms is even more striking for those who are hooking up for the first time. When Dr. Laurie Mintz anonymously polled her students at a large university for her book *Becoming Cliterate: Why Orgasm Equality Matters—and How to Get It*, she found that 55 percent of men versus only 4 percent of women reported reaching orgasm during first-time hookup sex.[2]

Most sexuality educators and researchers will agree that one of the main reasons there is a pleasure gap for women who have sex with men is that we live in a culture that overemphasizes penetrative vaginal intercourse and undervalues . . . everything else. Any sexual act other than penis-in-vagina sex is seen, by so many, as a less "real" form of sex. Unfortunately, this cultural ignorance of the importance of clitoral stimulation, which most people with vulvas require to reach an orgasm, has deep consequences for women's sexual pleasure when they partner with men.

Oral sex, vulva massage, stroking with fingers or toys, vibrator use on the clitoris—any of these acts increase the likelihood of an orgasm, but only the vulva owner knows for sure what works. Some women prefer anal penetration to vaginal, if they are to be penetrated at all. It is normal to require around twenty minutes of sexual attention to reach a level of arousal that makes vaginal penetration truly pleasurable.

The pleasure gap doesn't have to exist, and we know this because women who have sex with women rarely report gaps in pleasure. We do not currently have good data on trans, nonbinary, and gender-expansive pleasure, but we have decades upon decades of personal anecdotes, queer literature, queer films and media, and social media accounts that testify to the infinite ways queer and trans people find pleasure in their bodies. In other words, the pleasure gap seems to exist mostly in heterosexual-type relationships.

In the early stages of dating someone new, you and your partner will set up habits around your sexual connection, and you can take responsibility for creating habits that foster pleasure and open communication. Your partner is a full participant in creating those habits.

How comfortable do you feel talking with a new person about your sexual health? Do you know what you prefer when using barriers for STIs? If pregnancy prevention is important, what is the plan? How do they respond when you ask for a particular type of touch or sexual activity? How curious do they seem about your body and your pleasure? Being honest with yourself about these interactions early on is key to recognizing the patterns your sexual relationship might develop.

One of the first conversations to have with a new dating partner is about your sexual health practices and if you have any strong sexual preferences.

Here are a few practical tips for discussing sex with someone new.

1. Start the conversation before you are kissing, touching, or in bed.

2. Sit with some space between you, like at a table.

3. Allow your partner to choose to opt in to the conversation now, or to have it at another time. Some helpful conversation starters might be:

   • "I'd like to check in about our sexual health; is now a good time?"

   • "I like to talk about sex before it's happening; is that okay with you?"

   • "I'm excited for where this is going! Can we check in about a few things, like our safer sex practices and sexual preferences?"

4. Begin with the basics: Share your STI and testing status. Share your safer sex practice preferences. Share if you have other partners and whether you are using safer sex methods

with them so your new partner is aware of their level of risk and can make informed decisions.

If you know that you have strong sexual preferences—for example, you enjoy practicing BDSM and want a partner who can participate—share a bit about yourself. Then ask if there is anything else they want to know. Ask them to share a bit with you about the same topics.

5. Be kind to yourself no matter how it goes. Remember that sex cannot be ruined by open communication. It is okay to table the conversation for another time, at any point. You do not need to tell all your stories of sexual trauma to a new person. What you do need is to gauge their comfort with conversations about sexual topics and their capacity to listen for and respect boundaries.

6. Keep the door open. The goal here is sexual pleasure without fear. Perhaps you will need to negotiate boundaries around certain sexual activities or talk about what kind of sexual communication you both prefer. Ongoing communication is always preferable.

Falling in Love

You may be propelled into becoming more emotionally and sexually connected to another by the experience of falling in love. The feeling of falling for someone can make you feel very vulnerable. You may idealize your potential partner, seeing in them someone who can meet all your needs, who has the qualities you want, and who will be able to love you as you have always wanted to be loved.

Falling in love can feel like a longing to merge with your loved one, to become one in body and spirit. These experiences provide a heightened emotional and sexual connection. With this person you feel energized, excited, euphoric, on top of the world.

Once you become more connected to another person sexually and emotionally, you begin to know who that person really is. Usually at that point, the idealized image begins to fade away, and the real person becomes clearer to you.

Now comes a more mature choice. Ask yourself, "Is this someone I want to maintain a connection with? Is this someone I want to build a relationship with?" If you can honestly answer yes, then you can begin taking some calculated emotional risks. This is how you build the kind of intimate love relationship that will sustain and nurture you, by deepening your relationship in evolutionary stages.

Arati's Dating Dilemma

After dating a new person for a few months, Arati would usually find that she could not live without the euphoric feelings she had in the idealization stage of falling in love. She would find herself beginning to back away from the relationship when the idealization started to fade. She would tell herself it "wasn't meant to be" because her feelings had started to change.

Instead of choosing to build an intimate sexual relationship, she would go looking for someone else to fall in love with, and she would abandon the next relationship, too, as the initial euphoria faded into the attentiveness and decision-making required by authentic connection. For years, Arati dated new people, going from relationship to relationship, seeking those magical moments, in an addictive search for the high of being in love. Real intimacy never had time to develop. She used to tell herself that she would just know when it was right, and that she owed it to herself and her son not to settle for someone who didn't keep her happy.

Arati's most recent partner had ended their dating relationship before Arati ran away, which was a rare experience for her. She realized that she had not been able to show up fully to the relationship because of her out-of-control behaviors with alcohol and stimulant pills. She regretted not putting more care into the relationship, and she saw it as a chance for deeper intimacy that had been lost.

For a while, she tried to convince her ex-partner to try again. They told her they didn't see what would be different between them, and gently but firmly said no. Arati was hurt and angry, and she argued that her sobriety changed everything. Later, in therapy, Arati was able to accept that her ex-partner had made a decision, and that the most loving thing she could do was respect the boundary, allow herself to grieve, and take good care of herself.

Importantly, Arati realized that her sobriety hadn't changed everything after all. Her desire for the high of a new relationship was threaded throughout her life. Her difficulty trusting someone and allowing a relationship to grow was still present for her.

Now that she is focusing on her sobriety and self-pleasure, Arati feels more equipped to try dating again. She still has concerns about what it will look and feel like to build deeper intimacy with someone new. It scares her to imagine being consistently open, honest, vulnerable, and committed to someone, but it is a fear she'd like to face.

Miyu and Jake

Miyu had nearly a decade of recovery from disordered eating and three years of abstaining from self-harm under her belt when she first started dating again. At twenty-four, she felt she was lagging behind her peers and was terrified of sexual intimacy. Miyu's therapist referred her to a free online women's sexuality education group that met weekly. In the group, Miyu learned about basic anatomy, the impact of body image on sexual confidence, consent communication, and many other topics she had never heard discussed in school or at home. In her breakout group, she was able to process her feelings about dating a new person.

Almost immediately after their first few dates, Miyu began to lose herself in the intensity of falling for Jake. She put him at the center of her life. She stopped making plans with her friends unless she was sure Jake was unavailable. She was reprimanded at work for having her phone out during business hours too often, because she was texting with Jake. She felt extremely happy when she was with him, and terrible when they were apart. Sometimes they would argue, and Miyu would feel panicked. She would stay up all night on the phone with him to make sure he wasn't angry with her.

Miyu's essential identity became Jake's Girlfriend. How she felt about herself was a reflection of how Jake felt about her. In this process she sacrificed true intimacy for caretaking, placing someone else's needs in a primary place, often to the exclusion of her own. Jake enjoyed Miyu's company, in part because she was extremely attentive to his needs, wants, and desires. However, he soon grew less interested in her. Miyu had done everything she could think of to be an ideal girlfriend, but the relationship ended after several months. She was devastated. Nauseated and grief-stricken, Miyu returned to some disordered eating habits.

This woke her up. "I don't know how to love someone without disappearing," she told her peers at their weekly process group. They consoled her and offered her comfort.

"You deserve someone who is as interested in you as you are in him."

"You're amazing, and you're going to date someone who sees it too."

"Don't disappear! We missed you!"

"You got over a big fear to go out with him. I know it didn't work out, but I'm still proud of you."

With the help of her group, her therapist, and the years of recovery work she had already put in, Miyu tended to her grief after the breakup and returned to her healthier habits. She knew that she would try dating again when she felt stronger in herself, and she felt more patient now for love to grow over time with someone new.

The Risk of Sexual Intimacy

Learning to be comfortable in a new sexual relationship may take time. It will certainly require that you take emotional risks, and inevitably there will be bumps in the road.

You may find yourself feeling stuck in a relationship with a sexual partner who can't match you in a respectful, mutual, compassionate relationship. You may put your trust in people who eventually disappoint you. These situations will not be as devastating if you have developed a strong, grounded sense of intimacy with yourself and supportive friends.

Here are some questions you can ask yourself to determine if your sexual relationships have the capacity for intimacy:

- Do we have a sense of mutual respect?
- Do we have a mutual understanding about the level of emotional depth we want in our relationship?
- What happens when we have conflict? Do we work it out safely and with compassion? Do we assume good intentions from each other?
- Do I feel seen and understood? Do they indicate to me that they feel seen and understood?
- Do we support each other's growth?

- Are we honest with each other?
- Do we help each other reach our goals?
- Do I feel safe to be my full self with them?

Note that if you are nonmonogamous, you may have different answers to these questions for different partners. Perhaps you have identified a partner with whom you are not seeking deeper intimacy, but having a sexual and/or romantic connection with them is still enjoyable and fulfilling in your life. There are no rules that say every person has to achieve the highest level of intimacy possible to be a positive force in your life.

If you decide that your current sexual partner is someone with whom you'd like to become more intimate, you'll need to realize that doing so is a process that takes time. Some people plunge into sexual relationships hoping intimacy will follow, while others avoid being both intimate and sexual with the same person. Getting on the same page with your partner usually takes some effort.

In order to develop an intimate sexual relationship gradually, you will need to learn how to take calculated risks. That means taking a sexual or emotional risk that is appropriate to how vulnerable it makes you feel in that stage of the relationship. Begin with small risks that don't have enormous consequences if they don't work out. These will be different for everyone, but they could include sharing a fantasy with the person and seeing how they respond, calmly externalizing a disagreement with them about a small matter and noticing their reaction, letting them know that something they did or said was uncomfortable for you and discussing it with them, or sharing a favorite show, book, or movie with them.

This is not about calculation and strategy; it is about noticing opportunities to be honest, recognizing that there is some risk involved, and doing it anyway. Keep checking to make sure you're being honest with yourself, both emotionally and sexually.

You'll know you're in trouble if you start hiding your feelings, including your sexual feelings, from your partner. It is essential to be able to express your feelings and to be able to trust your partner to honor them rather than denigrate them. Ask yourself whether the relationship still feels respectful, mutual, and compassionate; whether you and your partner are giving and receiving at similar levels; and whether the relationship has gotten out of balance in any area.

Look at your level of trust. Is it growing? Or are you distancing and withdrawing? If the relationship continues to develop and deepen, then you can take greater emotional risks that require more vulnerability. Again, only you know which risks feel greater than others, but many people find that asking for help when they are struggling is a larger emotional risk. Other risks include spending time with each other's friends or families, asking for a conversation about how to increase your sexual pleasure with each other, and sharing more about your history with addiction or trauma and the efforts you are making now to heal and grow.

If you increase your level of vulnerability, your partner should be able to respond with increased vulnerability of their own. Watch out for imbalances. Ideally, you take trustworthy actions to care for each other after getting vulnerable. This in turn increases the level of intimacy you will feel.

Intimate Sexual Relationships

Being inside an intimate relationship is like being inside a warm home whose walls expand to encompass your growth. Within this relationship, you are free to express your vulnerability, to experience being truly seen and heard, and to become empathetic in both understanding and response. You and your partner act as mirrors for each other, reflecting each other's moods, thoughts, and actions. An intimate relationship can enable you to see yourself in a completely new way.

Intimacy takes place on a deep level. You are letting another person into a special place, letting yourself be seen and known. Becoming emotionally intimate with someone you are sexual with can be a frightening experience. Going the other direction, becoming sexual with someone you are already emotionally intimate with can be equally frightening. Notice, if you can, whether fear is leading you to act out in ways that violate your own values or integrity.

If you do feel afraid of or threatened by intimacy, like Arati discovered she did, you might respond by withdrawing or creating barriers between yourself and your sexual partner. You may distance yourself sexually, avoiding a deep sharing of your innermost self. Or you may allow yourself to share intimately while you're being sexual, but avoid vulnerability in your daily life.

You may find a certain level of intimacy comfortable in your sexual relationship, but panic when that relationship begins to grow and deepen. Notice if you feel compelled to test the strength of the relationship, to challenge your partner unnecessarily. Or, like Miyu, you may overextend into the relationship, becoming obsessed with the approval of your partner rather than getting closer with them.

If you were sexually abused as a child, you may have a particularly difficult time maintaining intimacy in sexual relationships. You will have to give yourself time to regain the capacity for trust and closeness that still lives within you, and remember that on the upward spiral of recovery and healing, you will still revisit some of the same issues from time to time.

It is also commonly said that people with substance use disorders have severe problems expressing intimacy. When you consider the impact of gender, the fear of intimacy that women, nonbinary people, and gender-expansive people may have is actually a well-grounded fear of emotional, physical, and sexual abuse. We know that women and girls from backgrounds that include out-of-control substance use are most likely to experience violence, abuse, and violation from those who have the closest proximity, like their friends, dating partners, and families. It is actually quite rational for women with substance use issues and/or prior traumatic experiences to fear intimacy; many have lived in situations in which their boundaries were violated by those who said "I love you."

The personal challenges you face to create an intimate loving relationship are not insurmountable. Please remain gentle with yourself as you navigate the complexity of becoming close with another person. As you learn more about your own tendencies, you can turn your loving attention to those parts of you that still ask for healing and support.

It is important to remember that people who have a history of trauma and addiction often enter relationships that also have addictive qualities. Intimacy is mutual, respectful, and compassionate—but obsession, loss of self in the other, and other forms of passionate romantic intensity can be easily mistaken for intimacy.

The following chart may help you sort out the differences between an intimate and an addictive relationship. If you are in a relationship now, consider which column feels more descriptive of your connection. If you are not in a relationship now, think of your most recent relationship or a significant relationship from your past.

Contrasting Intimate Relationships and Addictive Relationships

Here is a description of the qualities of a loving, intimate relationship versus those of an addictive relationship.

Intimate Relationship	Addictive Relationship
Mutuality (shared, balanced)	Power over (controlling behavior)
Choice	Loss of choice
Freedom	Compulsion
Honesty, openness	Avoiding truth, lying
Desire to share needs and feelings	No-talk rule, especially if things are not working out.
Relationship is able to include growth and change.	Relationship is always the same.
I want to be there.	I have to be there.
I begin with me (self).	I begin with you.
Can say "I want" and "I feel"	You make me feel . . .
Active, not passive	Reactive
I take care of me. I am solely responsible for figuring out what I need and for communicating it to you.	You will know what's right for me and you will fix it.
Relationship deals with reality.	Relationship is based on delusion/fantasy.
Relationship deals with things as they are, whatever comes along.	Relationship uses denial and avoidance to deal with things.
I have a true interest in your personal/spiritual growth, even if it takes you away from me.	Your spiritual growth doesn't count.
Love is always an act of self-love.	Love is wanting someone with me at all costs.

Source: Adaptation of the text from pages 180–181 of *Leaving the Enchanted Forest* by Stephanie Covington and Liana Beckett. Copyright © 1988 by Stephanie Covington and Liana Beckett. Reprinted by permission of HarperCollins Publishers.

One quality of many addictive relationships that makes them difficult to let go of is their passion. The intensity of feeling that can accompany addictive relationships is easily mistaken for love. And sometimes that passion and desire to be together can be transformed from an addictive experience into a relationship that is nourishing and intimate, but both parties must take responsibility and do the emotional work to make it so.

Vanessa likes to call intimate relationships "low-drama love," and says of a current partner, "we don't have that kind of desperately hot makeup sex because we don't have the same desperately lonely, horrible fights. Sometimes I miss that kind of sex, but I don't miss the suffering. Sexual desire is different from this place. It moves slower, emerges from deeper within my body. Low-drama love requires deliberate action toward sexual connection. The difference is that sexual creativity is such a gorgeous playground when you are safe to play."

If sexual desire and passion seemed easier to access in the past, know that you are not alone. Intimate sexual relationships create sexual connection from a foundation of safety, not confusion or danger, and this can take time to build or adjust to. Many people associate sexual feelings with stress, and our bodies respond powerfully to those associations.

It can help to remember that there are more types of sexual intimacy than any of us can imagine! You may have slow, sensual, eye-gazing lovemaking at one time, then raunchy, loud, messy sex another time, and any of the other infinite options as well. The key is that you trust your partner to show up with the intention of creating pleasure together, and you hold that intention as well. The exploration of what that means on any given day is yours to enjoy.

○ ◉ ○

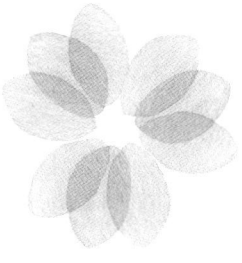

CHAPTER 12

The Continuing Journey of Sexual Recovery

As a culture, we often confuse or have a limited idea of what pleasure is. I want to expand the idea of what pleasure is and highlight the tool and guide that it can be. Pleasure is not always something that, from beginning to end, makes us feel happy. If we look at pleasure in a more expansive way, pleasure can also mean contentment, satisfaction, quiet calmness, the fierce rush of internal movement toward coherence, or outward struggle against an adversary or challenge.... When we're committed to healing, committed to growth, committed to connection, and committed to pleasure there can be a kind of pleasure in doing anything.

Jamila Dawson, *With Pleasure: Managing Trauma Triggers for More Vibrant Sex and Relationships,* co-authored with August McLaughlin

Recovery is about expansion. It is about awakening to all that
is possible in life. It is about integrating your inner life and
your outer life, so that what's happening on the inside—your
values, your beliefs, and your feelings—are being represented in
your outer life, in your actions with other people in the world.
If your inner and outer lives are consistent, coherent, and con-
gruent, you will experience integrity. For many, this integrity is
the foundation of their spirituality.

Remember, we use the word *spirituality* as loosely as possible,
to gesture at whatever way you stay connected to something
greater than yourself. When talking about pleasure, sex, and relationships, we can easily forget that our most intimate, personal,
and intense feelings are actually part of the larger world around
us. Not only are we connected to all who have lived, loved, experienced pain, struggled with addiction, or survived trauma before
us, but we are connected to thousands who are experiencing
something similar in their own lives right now.

Your sexuality is unique to you, and at the same time, it is
part of what connects you to the world, people, environment,
and social forces around you. Imagined this way, sexuality is
inextricable from the energy of being alive.

We sometimes feel, and rightly so, that we have been trained to give up our sexuality in order to be more spiritual. Patriarchal religions dictate that our sexuality must be controlled by strict moral codes, and often reserved only for procreation. But what if we proceed from the belief that sexuality and spirituality are interconnected? They are both about the life force that is within us. They have enormous capacity to enrich our lives.

How you express your sexuality is your choice. If you choose to share your sexual self with another person, you are responsible for what you create together. Sexuality is a creative force, and you get to decide what kind of energy, relationship, or experience you want to bring into the world with your focused, present-moment attention. This chapter continues our discussion of intimacy, love, and deeper connections, with the goal of opening new directions for you in your ongoing recovery.

The Challenge of Safety

One of the most profound human experiences is to be intimate with another human being. To know and be known, to see and be seen, to understand and be understood: This is intimacy with another. It can take a great deal of effort to create intimacy with yourself, and intimacy with others requires even more care. Emotional safety is the foundation of intimacy, and many of us struggle to find, build, or feel it.

A major challenge is living in a society that does not provide an environment conducive to intimacy. No one can ignore the real-life situations we live in, from which our relationships emerge. One example is how many relationships are affected by financial hardship—some feel stuck with a partner because they can't afford to leave, while others break up over money concerns.

Challenges to safety and intimacy emerge based on who is involved in the relationship, where, and when. Gender, sexual orientation, age, disability, and so many more parts of who we are affect our relationships and how we create intimacy with others.

In her introduction to *Disability Intimacy: Essays on Love, Care, and Desire*, disability rights activist Alice Wong reminds us that most discourse surrounding intimacy and disability is disappointingly simplistic, if not outright offensive. As a person who uses a wheelchair, Wong has been on the receiving end of American stigma and misinformation about the desires of disabled people since she was a child. Wong writes, "Not everyone needs romance or sex, but I personally want the entire dim sum cart of intimacy. I want to experience every unctuous, savory, sweet, crispy, chewy, spicy, and sour bite, filling my body with warmth and pleasure."[1]

The challenges to intimate relationships come from both the outside and the inside. This means intimacy is created by those who want to do the outer and inner work. Wong identifies tenderness as a theme among the stories in *Disability Intimacy*—a quality most relationships need more of. But tenderness is something we express most easily when we are feeling safe, and safety must be built through deliberate actions of care. If this sounds circular, remember the upward spiral. We return to the work of tending our relationships time and again.

Our healing begins with ourselves, but it can truly blossom only through connection with another person or people. If trauma happened in a relationship, then ultimately we need to feel a safe connection with other people to heal. We may grieve the end of our relationship with someone who harmed us, but then how do we learn to trust again?

We must address the specific challenges that arise for each one of us. Understanding our challenges, we see what we can do to communicate honestly, listen wholeheartedly, and navigate toward a deeper understanding and connection with the people in our lives now.

For Those Who Partner with Men

Relationships that have more social support are not immune to the struggle for safety. Our culture is supportive of heterosexual-type relationships, and yet, women who identify as primarily heterosexual often have problems creating emotional safety, tenderness, and intimacy with the men they choose as partners. Much of this is directly related to gender differences in American socialization in childhood and beyond.

The instructions for "being a man" include this rule: Don't express feelings of confusion, weakness, fear, vulnerability, tenderness, compassion, and sensuality. It makes sense, then, that many men struggle to feel comfortable with intimacy.

Many men develop powerful denial systems that allow them to block out unwelcome feelings, which are exactly the ones women find they miss in their partners. The qualities that American men are encouraged to embody, such as aggression, competition, independence, control, and decisiveness, are of limited value in forming and maintaining intimate relationships. As women recognize the limits of their own socialization, relationships with men can become more problematic and less satisfying.

In the words of one woman in recovery who was recently widowed, "Everybody always remarked on how well we got along. We never fought. But the reason we got along so well was that I did everything he wanted, like the good little wife. Now I feel like I have a chance to get myself back."

Men's socialization in the area of explicit sexual behavior creates another sort of problem. Men are socialized to be in charge sexually, to be aggressive, to make the moves and risk rejection. They might work hard to learn how to perform sexually, and they can feel as if they are responsible for making sex happen. This goal-oriented drive to penetrative intercourse, ejaculation, and orgasm, and an accompanying lack of attention to sex of any other kind, can leave women feeling deprioritized, angry, and frustrated. The proliferation of jokes and memes about men not knowing how to find the clitoris strikes many women as funny because the jokes hint at a truth about the gap in men's and women's pleasure.

Of course, the positive scenario is also possible! As women work to become able to ask for what they want sexually, they may find that the men they date are turned on by their increased assertiveness. Some men feel deep relief when allowing themselves to receive sexual attention that does not require them to "perform," and they have genuine curiosity about women's bodies and pleasure. While dating men, you may find that just as you are working to change and grow sexually, many men are too.

After working so hard to break out of our own inauthentic sexual behavior to experience who we really are, we don't want to go back to performing a sexual role that we didn't choose. Connecting with men who are ready to explore a more creative, unique, and nontraditional way of connecting sexually is possible. It may be challenging, but they want to find you as badly as you want to find them.

As Michelle continued in therapy, she began to talk more about Chris, and specifically about all the ways in which he wasn't perfect. She wanted him to be more communicative, to share his feelings, but he seemed to be resisting. He was glad that Michelle maintained sobriety from alcohol and pills, but he became a little confused by the changes in their relationship. In couple's therapy, they tried to address new issues as they came up.

Although Chris loves Michelle and has stayed with her through some very difficult years of out-of-control drinking and early recovery, her former emotional unavailability and the fact that she made few emotional demands on him actually worked for him rather well. The chaos of her life contrasted with his reliability and dependability. This dynamic made him feel powerful and in control.

In recovery, however, Michelle wants a more flexible, spontaneous, generous partner. It is a major adjustment, and it asks more of Chris than he originally imagined. He had not planned to be in therapy just for himself, but their couple's therapist suggested he may need more support than he is getting.

Michelle is beginning to know herself as a sexual person in her own right and has some sexual needs and desires of her own. She wants to be held and touched; she wants affection without sex. She also wants Chris to focus on her sexual pleasure and enjoy doing so. She wants to be creative sexually, without the pressure of whether or not he gets an erection affecting them both so much.

Chris will have to step up to a new way of creating sexual and emotional intimacy in the marriage. This may be a big challenge, but he has shown himself to be courageous in the face of Michelle's major changes before. Michelle will need to remember to be patient with Chris's pace of change. She can refocus on her own body and pleasure whenever she is starting to obsessively try to make Chris change.

For Those Who Partner with Women, Nonbinary People, and Gender-Expansive People

While some queer relationships deal with similar issues to heterosexual relationships, especially when it comes to substance use disorders and addictive behaviors, many also face some quite different challenges. Research suggests that lesbian women do not complain primarily about relationship problems in communicating, tenderness, or sexual performance. The greatest problems seem to stem from living in a culture that is unsupportive of lesbian identity, and the significantly higher rates of poverty for LGBTQ+ people.

American society's tremendous bias toward heterosexuality and corresponding negativity toward gay, lesbian, bisexual, and other queer sexual identities, is still quite robust. Add in cultural bias against polyamorous relationships and other types of nonmonogamy, sexual subcultures including kink and leather communities, and any other sexuality considered nonnormative. Now consider the many ways we can feel and express gender, especially trans, nonbinary, and gender-expansive expression. For queer people, there are many intersecting stigmas affecting relationship health.

First and most important is honesty with yourself and reducing as much shame as you can about your desires, preferences, body, orientation, or identity. Gently remind yourself that sexual variety is the most normal thing in the world. Queer relationships can thrive in safer communities. The work of intimacy may require addressing internalized stigma or processing the pain of oppressive people and systems. Examples of queer love, joy, and sex are important to the collective experience.

For All

Many people use mood-altering substances or addictive behaviors as a mediator between sexual behavior or desire and self-acceptance. Without those habits that numb us, we will encounter our past sexual histories and current sexual desires directly. These encounters can be deeply challenging. Some may have anesthetized their sexual feelings in fear of them; others may have been able to be sexual only when high or drunk.

No matter the partner or relationship style, you need to have a safe place in which to explore your sexual feelings and needs. Individual therapy and groups for women and nonbinary people who are investigating their sexuality can be particularly helpful during this time.

When looking for a support group or therapist, make sure to test the waters to find out if your whole self will be welcome. Are you interested in a women-only group? Is a group inclusive of nonbinary, trans, and other queer members? Does the practitioner list "LGBTQ+-friendly" on their website? Is there a trained sex therapist available? Are all love styles and relationship configurations welcome at this meetup? Is this a body- and disability-inclusive space? Even if you don't carry a specific marginalized identity, you may look for these signs to ensure that you are entering a more inclusive space.

Conscious Love and Commitment

Joyce was in her mid-forties when she entered therapy with co-author Stephanie. She had been in recovery from alcohol use disorder for two years, as had her husband, Howard. They had been married for twenty years and had two boys, both in their late teens. For the last ten years of marriage, Joyce and Howard had not been sexual with each other.

The first time Stephanie met Joyce, she seemed burdened. She was neatly dressed, but her shoulders sagged. She was ready to talk, and her story came tumbling out. "My husband has an erectile problem; we haven't had sex for ten years. I'm in recovery, and I'm living my life really fully. But this piece is missing, and I don't know if I want to remain married knowing we're never going to have sex again." They no longer touched; they were distant friends living in the same house but never connecting.

Stephanie wasn't sure how she could help. Even if Howard's erectile dysfunction was not a medical issue, his performance anxiety and fears after such a long time would be significant. Stephanie decided to aim not toward sexual performance, but toward building trust. She hoped to help the couple develop a feeling of closeness and intimacy.

Periodically, Joyce would tell Howard what was going on in therapy. He felt very protective about his own sexual history and was threatened and intimidated by his wife being in therapy. Many times, he poohpoohed it, saying, "No one has any business knowing about our sex life." He was not an active and willing participant in the process.

Eventually Stephanie asked Joyce to list all the sensual activities she wanted to experience with her husband. Then she was asked to list them again in the order of things that would be easiest to ask for. Each activity was to remain discrete: They were never to proceed further. For example, if he gave her a back rub, he was to confine his touching to her back only. In addition, only positive feedback could be given.

Then it was time to try the list on Howard. Joyce started with the least difficult, asking him to give her a back rub. His initial response to the back rub was, "This is ridiculous, what's the big deal about this?" Joyce replied, "This is something I really want to do." So he rubbed her back, she said it felt good, and he just sort of grumbled.

The next week she had him rub her back again, but now with body oil. This time when she said it felt good, he said, "Oh, well, this does feel better." Stephanie was encouraged. This was the first clue that Howard had feeling or sensation in his body and that he could admit to Joyce that somehow it felt better to touch her body with oil. So Howard *did* feel, and what he was feeling could be accessed more easily than Stephanie had initially thought.

Several weeks later, Joyce took a shower with Howard. It only lasted a minute, but they did it. Then a few more weeks later, they took a bath together, and eventually, they enjoyed a bubble bath, with music and candles. Throughout this months-long process, Howard never had an erection. But as they went through the list of activities, something more important began to happen: They found themselves having spontaneous moments of connection, separate from the exercises.

Sometimes, while they were watching television, he would reach out and hold her hand. When they went to bed, he would cuddle up close. When he said goodbye in the morning, there was a different quality to the hug and kiss. Joyce began to feel differently about Howard, more connected. At times, she was very touched and moved by his spontaneous expressions of affection. The quality of their connection had begun to improve.

Even though their activities were externally focused, what they were working on was internal change. Joyce realized that she had been missing not only physical contact but some kind of closeness and intimacy. And this was now returning to their relationship.

The last thing on Joyce's list was oral sex. After nearly a year of slowly creating more intimacy, she asked him if he wanted to try. To Joyce's surprise, Howard was amenable to the idea and even a little excited about it. Joyce had an orgasm, and Howard was absolutely delighted. He got a great deal of pleasure out of giving her pleasure. As a result, something really changed for him. It was a very powerful moment. Somehow this man, who had not been sexually active for ten years, had brought his wife to a point of real pleasure, and he was very moved by that experience.

Soon after that, Joyce stopped going to therapy with Stephanie. About six months later, she called. She was laughing. "You're not going to believe what happened. Howard just called me and said he was on his way home and he had made his own list of things he wanted to experience with me!"

Maybe Joyce and Howard returned to having intercourse, and maybe not. The most encouraging part of their story is how they were able to reconnect and have a satisfying relationship without it.

Sex in any particular form is not the ultimate goal of sexuality, but it is one important facet in a complex expression of our whole being. For Joyce and Howard, the choice to continue showing each other love opened the door for a renewed interested in their sexual connection.

In conscious love, you choose to be with each other, to build a relationship together over time. Choice is crucial to conscious love: The power and capacity to choose is what makes your intimacy authentic, and exercising that ability is basic to your recovery.

Passionate love can bring us together. It's that longing for union with another, a bridge to end our separation, a longing for connection. When intimacy and authentic sexual expression merge in one relationship, you will make a profound connection. But it may not look the way you expect. The experience of falling in love can be the prelude to an expansive and growth-fostering experience: the ongoing practice of choosing conscious love.

In choosing conscious love, you also choose mature interdependence. You allow yourself truly to connect with and depend on your partner, but you retain your autonomy of self. You choose a partner who values your recovery and who also chooses to engage in the process with you. They are in a process of their own, and you mutually support each other's growth.

Choosing to be together is making a commitment. A loving commitment is not about the length of time you've been together; many of us know couples who have stayed together, without respect or mutuality, for decades. It is also not necessarily about monogamy or planning far into the future—these may or may not be aspects of a commitment, and they do not define it.

Loving commitment is about choosing to be there; to be intimate, open, and vulnerable; to do your best to be available to the other person while attending also to yourself. Loving commitment will allow you to feel safe and secure, knowing that the other person has also chosen to be open, available, and vulnerable. Loving commitment requires choosing this not once, but again and again. The value of authentic, intimate sexual relationships is in their power to heal and change us. They empower us and cause us to grow.

Many people feel uncertain about what form of commitment is viable in their own lives. You may view your commitment to your work as both liberating and exciting, for example, but see possible commitment to a partner as limiting and restricting. You may long to fall back on lifelong vows that are unrelated to your changing needs and wants, because it feels safer to play a role rather than be your authentic self. You may reach middle age longing for the stability that a twenty-year relationship can bring, concerned about the seven-year average of American marriages. We are all going to have some concerns about love and commitment, and the concerns may feel overwhelming.

Still, the work is to be done in the present moment. Being committed means that you have promised to engage in a process with yourself and, if possible, your partner. The key is your willingness to be present with each other through the changes in your lives. You can learn to move into relationships gradually, both emotionally and physically.

It is possible for those in long-term relationships to lose intimacy but to regain it anew. Some partners who have been together for years in a distanced or conflicted relationship may need to start their relationship all over again. They may need to relearn basic elements of sensuality and intimacy, such as how to hold hands, how to sit close on the sofa, how to experience the pleasure of each other's skin. Slowly, bit by bit, the levels of emotional and physical intimacy and connection can deepen. In the words of Ev'Yan Whitney, author of *Sensual Self: Prompts and Practices for Getting in Touch with Your Body*, "It's a beautiful serendipity that by reclaiming and embodying our sensuality, we are better able to reclaim and embody our sexuality."[2]

Ecstasy Is Real

Actor, author, and activist Gillian Anderson put out a call for women to send her their sexual fantasies, anonymously, for a book. The result is *Want: Women's Fantasies in the Twenty-First Century*, a collection of hundreds of fantasies from women and nonbinary people across the world—religious, atheist, rich, poor, middle class, married to men, married to women, cisgender, transgender, single, cohabiting, with and without children—the diversity of voices and variety of sexual imaginings on display in *Want* is remarkable. Among many important provocations, Anderson asks: "If we could loosen the chains of shame out in the real world, what new, pleasurable heights might we all be able to reach?"[3]

Those "pleasurable heights" are a state of being that is often called *ecstasy*. (It's no coincidence that a drug of the same name floods your body with pleasurable sensation!)

Author and educator Dr. Emily Nagoski has asked hundreds of people what benefit the feeling of ecstasy has had in their lives. Overwhelmingly, they answer that it brings them connection: with a partner, with themselves, and with something larger than themselves. Nagoski calls arriving at ecstasy "the magic trick." Others call it an experience of "the universe," "the divine," "Spirit," "infinity," and so on.

Ecstatic sexual experience is one way for us to stay fully in the present moment and to appreciate how expansive it is. It does not usually happen by accident or without the work of real connection. In being sexual, we can meld with the other, losing the boundary of skin to skin, and exist in a sort of timelessness. Sometimes sexual ecstasy can even be our introduction to an authentic spiritual dimension in ourselves.

Tamara had left her Christian upbringing behind when she came out as a lesbian in her late teens. The rupture with her family, especially her mother, was difficult. As far as Tamara was concerned, many decades later, spirituality had been a coercive force in her life, and she was not interested in reconnecting with it. However, she kept encountering people who believed that some form of spirituality was a crucial aspect of recovery. Then she learned about the connection between mindfulness meditation and chronic pain, did some research, and decided to try it.

She told her therapist that she had begun to sit in silence for a few minutes each day. "I don't sit on a cushion because of my back pain," she said. "I sit in a chair. I sometimes fall asleep. But I keep trying to just find a quiet place inside."

Tamara read articles about Black spiritual leaders like the Buddhist and civil rights activist Alvin Sykes. She turned her powerful curiosity toward the myriad ways Black Americans embodied spirituality, and she found many who had chosen the path of meditation. This emboldened her in her mindfulness practice.

She signed up for a women's weekend meditation retreat, mostly on a whim.

Unexpectedly, she had an incredible time. She later shared with her recovery group that she had meditated for hours each day, sometimes in silence, sometimes walking, sometimes listening to teachings. Tamara found that while meditating, every now and then she could actually feel energy moving up and down her body, sometimes collecting in one place, other times staying in flow.

Another wonderful thing happened at that retreat: Tamara met someone she felt attracted to. Over the last dinner of the weekend, Tamara found out that Lucy enjoyed her company too, and they began to spend time together back home. Their relationship developed slowly, with a deep foundation of mutual respect and friendship.

Tamara was joyful for the first time in a long time. When she and Lucy were sexual, it was unlike any other experience she had had. "Sometimes when I'm with Lucy," she says, "I'm feeling something bigger than our physical bodies. I can't control when it is going to happen, although it's pretty clear when it won't—my pain is flaring up, or the stress of the day is too much. But when we are able to really relax into our intimacy, it sometimes feels like we are floating together, not two separate people, and I have this incredible sensation of warmth that envelops us."

This wonderful new experience came with some grief for Tamara, as she faced the reality that she had never been this vulnerable or present with Alisha, her ex-wife. At the same time,

Tamara and Lucy, both in their sixties, rarely had the kind of spontaneous, urgent sex Alisha and Tamara had enjoyed in their forties.

"I'm learning to let go of my expectations," Tamara says. "Of course, I hope that I'll continue to have these sorts of experiences—both in sex and in meditation—but I've let go of them as goals. I love touching Lucy and being touched by her. Bonding with her feels special and precious. And if sometimes we enter another level of consciousness together, well," she smiles, "I'll take that gift."

For Tamara, sexuality and spirituality became an integrated whole, without her needing to have all the answers.

Embracing the Pleasure of Change

Let's revisit a few important questions about sexuality as we reach our conclusion. As you answer these for yourself, recall how you may have answered them differently while you read chapter 1, versus now.

- What does it mean to become a sexual person in our society?
- What does it mean to have this complex thing called sexuality integrated into our lives in a meaningful way?
- What is your own unique experience of pleasure, and how do you cultivate it in a way that makes you feel glad to be alive?

Perhaps you have a clearer, more nuanced way to address these questions now that you have progressed along your own upward spiral of sexual recovery. We can add some new questions to the mix, adapted from Euphemia Russell's book *Slow Pleasure: Explore Your Pleasure Spectrum*:

What do you think a pleasure-based culture would look like and feel like? How would it look beyond the individual experience of pleasure? Beyond the experience of expressed pleasure with lovers and partners? How would a pleasure-based culture be inter-relational and communal?[4]

Our interconnectedness is undeniable. Our ability to feel pleasure in the midst of chaotic circumstances, difficulty, and change is key to our resilience and connection to others. Sexuality is not fixed; it is a part of you that will change with you as you change. Embracing the pleasure of change begins with knowing where we have been, and appreciating where we are now.

The following twelve messages are drawn from the chapters you have just read and are offered here and as note cards at the end of this chapter to take with you as you move along your upward spiral of recovery and healing.

1. It is possible for you to face what is unknown or painful about your own sexuality and grow into a new, loving relationship with this part of yourself.

2. What we seek is self-awareness, so we can be fully at choice whenever we are sexual.

3. No matter how much or how little spontaneous desire you feel, your unique sexuality can respond to pleasure.

4. You can live in a deeper state of acceptance, even gratitude, for your body, exactly as it is right now.

5. Looking honestly at your sexual past is essential to sexual recovery. Sometimes you will need a boost of courage to look at the reality of your life. Sometimes you will need permission to go slowly, rest, and recuperate.

6. It is normal to have some trouble identifying and asserting sexual limits and boundaries, because it is normal to have had insufficient or even harmful education about sexuality.

7. It is as important to take a long, careful look at your partners' behavior as it is to look at your own behavior. This is not because you can change them, but because you can see where you need to adjust your own boundaries and communication.

8. When you feel powerless, you can seek support. When you feel powerful, you can offer strength and support to yourself and others. An ebb and flow is to be expected.

9. Sexuality can become creative, a source of energy and interest, rather than a place of fear or numbness.

10. As we move toward establishing real intimacy in our lives, it becomes clear that intimacy with ourselves is our foundation for intimacy with others.

11. A great sexual relationship is nourishing, sustaining, pleasurable, and growth-fostering. It takes skill to maintain. The first skill is friendship.

12. Ongoing recovery is a process that circles around similar issues like an upward spiral. The work to be done is in the present moment, and as we move through our changes, more options for pleasure, connection, and intimacy open up.

As you decide what is next for you, we encourage you to take a few moments to fully celebrate the effort you put into awakening your sexuality. In a time of profound isolation, shame, and the normalization of hatred, the creation of loving connections with ourselves and others becomes ever more important.

Sexuality can be such a powerful force in our lives, and it is all our responsibility to face the personal past and make decisions now that reflect our desires and our integrity.

Our wish for you: When you are engaged in sexual connection, with yourself or others, may it be a source of joy for you. Enjoy the richness and variety of your unique sexuality as you grow and change over time. Your sensuality, eroticism, and sexuality can be a force for good.

○ ○ ○

NOTE CARDS

It is possible for you to face what is
unknown or painful about your own sexuality
and grow into a new, loving relationship
with this part of yourself.

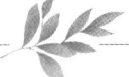

What we seek is self-awareness,
so we can be fully at choice
whenever we are sexual.

No matter how much or how little
spontaneous desire you feel, your unique
sexuality can respond to pleasure.

You can live in a deeper state of acceptance, even gratitude, for your body, exactly as it is right now.

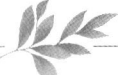

Looking honestly at your sexual past is essential to sexual recovery. Sometimes you will need a boost of courage to look at the reality of your life. Sometimes you will need permission to go slowly, rest, and recuperate.

It is normal to have some trouble identifying and asserting sexual limits and boundaries, because it is normal to have had insufficient or even harmful education about sexuality.

It is as important to take a long, careful look at your partners' behavior as it is to look at your own behavior. This is not because you can change them, but because you can see where you need to adjust your own boundaries and communication.

When you feel powerless, you can seek support. When you feel powerful, you can offer strength and support to yourself and others. An ebb and flow is to be expected.

Sexuality can become creative, a source of energy and interest, rather than a place of fear or numbness.

As we move toward establishing real intimacy in our lives, it becomes clear that intimacy with ourselves is our foundation for intimacy with others.

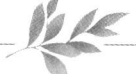

A great sexual relationship is nourishing, sustaining, pleasurable, and growth-fostering. It takes skill to maintain. The first skill is friendship.

Ongoing recovery is a process that circles around similar issues like an upward spiral. The work to be done is in the present moment, and as we move through our changes, more options for pleasure, connection, and intimacy open up.

NOTES

CHAPTER 2

1. Aubrey Gordon, *"You Just Need to Lose Weight" and 19 Other Myths About Fat People* (Beacon, 2023), 50.
2. Gordon, *"You Just Need to Lose Weight,"* 9.
3. "100 Women: 'I Transitioned and Lost My Male Privilege,'" BBC News, October 4, 2017, accessed July 22, 2024, https://www.bbc.com/news/av/world-41502661.

CHAPTER 3

1. Emily Nagoski, *Come As You Are: The Surprising New Science That Will Transform Your Sex Life* (Simon & Schuster, 2021), 42–69.
2. L. Froehle et al., "Bacterial Vaginosis and Alcohol Consumption: A Cross-Sectional Retrospective Study in Baltimore, Maryland," *Sexually Transmitted Diseases* 48, no. 12 (December 2021): 986–90, https://journals.lww.com/stdjournal/abstract/2021/12000/bacterial_vaginosis_and_alcohol_consumption__a.15.aspx.
3. Info NMN, "Patterns of Stress and Resilience," Neurosequential Network Stress and Trauma Series, 2020, accessed July 2024, https://www.youtube.com/watch?v=orwIn02h6V4&list=PLyhWK71WKiZKVixTQ3fFI-exZK29v_4iF.

CHAPTER 4

1. Sonya Renee Taylor, *The Body Is Not an Apology: The Power of Radical Self-Love,* 2nd ed. (Berret-Koehler, 2021), 4.

2. Andee Tagle and Clare Marie Schneider, "Diet Culture Is Everywhere. Here's How to Fight It," National Public Radio, January 4, 2022, accessed July 2024, https://www.npr.org /2021/12/23/1067210075/what-if-the-best-diet-is-to-reject -diet-culture.

3. Carla S. Alvarado, Diane M. Cassidy, Kendal Orgera, and Sarah Piepenbrink, "Polling Spotlight: Understanding the Experiences of LGBTQ+ Birthing People," AAAMC Center for Health Justice, June 27, 2022, accessed July 31, 2024, https://www .aamchealthjustice.org/news/polling/lgbtq-birth.

4. Jessi Kneeland, *Body Neutral: A Revolutionary Guide to Overcoming Body Image Issues* (Penguin, 2023), 32.

CHAPTER 6

1. Douglas Braun-Harvey and Michael A. Vigorito, *Treating Out of Control Sexual Behavior: Rethinking Sex Addiction* (Springer, 2016), 28.

CHAPTER 8

1. Elise Gould, "Gender Wage Gap Persists in 2023: Women Are Paid Roughly 22% Less Than Men on Average," Economic Policy Institute, Working Economics Blog, March 8, 2024, accessed September 30, 2024, https://www.epi.org/blog/gender-wage -gap-persists-in-2023-women-are-paid-roughly-22-less-than -men-on-average.

CHAPTER 9

1. Roxane Gay, *Not That Bad: Dispatches from Rape Culture* (Harper Perennial, 2018), ii.
2. Office of Justice Programs, "Responding to Transgender Victims of Sexual Assault," June 2014, accessed October 15, 2024, https://ovc.ojp.gov/sites/g/files/xyckuh226/files/pubs/forge /sexual_numbers.html.
3. VAWnet, "Marital Rape: New Research and Directions," February 2006, accessed October 15, 2024, https://vawnet.org /material/marital-rape-new-research-and-directions.
4. Amy Vorenberg, Jessica Durkis-Stokes, and Jessica C. Brown, *Utmost Resistance: Examining Sexual Violence Law in the United States* (Carolina Academic Press, 2024), 122.

CHAPTER 10

1. Lori A. Brotto, *Better Sex Through Mindfulness: How Women Can Cultivate Desire* (Greystone, 2018), 237.

CHAPTER 11

1. Laurie Mintz, *Becoming Cliterate: Why Orgasm Matters— and How to Get It* (HarperOne, 2017), 8.
2. Mintz, *Becoming Cliterate*, 9.

CHAPTER 12

1. Alice Wong, *Disability Intimacy: Essays on Love, Care, and Desire* (Vintage, 2024), xix.
2. Ev'Yan Whitney, *Sensual Self: Prompts and Practices for Getting in Touch with Your Body* (Clarkson Potter, 2021), 10.
3. Gillian Anderson, *Want: Women's Fantasies in the Twenty-First Century* (Abrams, 2024), 90.
4. Euphemia Russell, *Slow Pleasure: Explore Your Pleasure Spectrum* (Hardie Grant, 2022), 212.

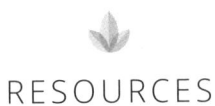

RESOURCES

Recovery Groups and Therapists

Please note: Some of these resources are free, and others have a membership fee or other cost. We list them here to offer you options to explore, not to recommend any particular program. If a program is based in the Twelve Step model developed by Alcoholics Anonymous, it will be noted.

LifeRing Secular Recovery
https://lifering.org/

Abstinence-based anonymous, secular meetings. Online and in person. All genders. No cost.

The Luckiest Club
https://www.theluckiestclub.com/

Dogma-free, compassionate place to recover from alcohol addiction and thrive in life. Online. All genders, with women's, LGBTQIA2S+, and BIPOC-only meetings. Monthly membership fee.

Manhattan Alternative
https://www.manhattanalternative.com/

Kink, poly, trans, and LGBTQ+-affirmative mental health providers. National online directory. Providers' fees will vary.

Moderation Management
https://moderation.org/

Behavior change program and peer-led support groups.
Online. All genders. No cost.

Psychology Today Therapist Finder
https://www.psychologytoday.com/us

Online directory of individual therapists and support groups.
Cost varies.

Sex and Love Addicts Anonymous (SLAA)
https://slaafws.org/

Online portal for the Twelve Step, Twelve Traditions–oriented
fellowship (based on AA model) for those who desire to stop
living out a pattern of sex and love addiction. Online and
in-person meetings. Open to all, with gender-specific meetings available. No cost.

SHE RECOVERS Foundation
https://sherecovers.org/

Nonprofit movement for women. Online and facilitated
groups, gatherings, and professional training. For women and
nonbinary individuals, with meetings specific to LGBTQ+,
BIPOC, veterans, mothers, and more. Meetings are free;
other costs vary based on service.

The Small Bow
https://www.thesmallbow.com/

Newsletter, podcast, and online recovery meetings.
All genders. Cost varies from free to subscription.

SMART Recovery
https://smartrecovery.org/

Evidence-informed approach to overcoming addictive behaviors. Online and in person. All genders. No cost.

Wombat Mental Health Services (for CA residents only)
https://wombatmhs.com/

Therapist-matching service providing equitable access to culturally appropriate, nonjudgmental, and affirmative mental health services for individuals from communities who have historically faced barriers in accessing care. All genders. Telehealth. Costs vary based on service and provider.

Women for Sobriety
https://womenforsobriety.org/

Peer-support program for women overcoming substance use disorders (SUDs). Online and in person. Women, nonbinary, and gender-expansive. No cost.

Sexuality, Bodies, and Pleasure

Allbodies
https://allbodies.com/

Online health classes that address sex, mental health, body literacy, and social justice. Costs vary per class.

OMGYES
https://www.omgyes.com/

Online library of instructional videos created from the largest research study into women's pleasure. Onetime payment for access to the library.

Planned Parenthood

https://www.plannedparenthood.org/learn/for-educators/
digital-tools

Free sexuality education resources.

Books

*Becoming Cliterate: Why Orgasm Equality Matters—and How
to Get It* by Laurie Mintz (HarperOne, 2017)

*Better Sex Through Mindfulness: How Women Can Cultivate
Desire* by Lori A. Brotto (Greystone Books, 2018)

The Body Is Not an Apology: The Power of Radical Self-Love,
2nd ed., by Sonya Renee Taylor (Berrett-Koehler, 2021)

*Body Neutral: A Revolutionary Guide to Overcoming Body Image
Issues* by Jessi Kneeland (Penguin Random House, 2023)

*Come As You Are: The Surprising New Science That Will Trans-
form Your Sex Life* by Emily Nagoski, PhD (Simon & Schuster,
2021)

Disability Intimacy: Essays on Love, Care, and Desire edited
by Alice Wong (Vintage, 2024)

Pleasure Activism: The Politics of Feeling Good edited by
adrienne maree brown (AK Press, 2019)

*Refusing Compulsory Sexuality: A Black Asexual Lens on Our
Sex-Obsessed Culture* by Sherronda J. Brown (North Atlantic
Books, 2022)

*Sensual Self: Prompts and Practices for Getting in Touch with
Your Body* by Ev'Yan Whitney (Clarkson Potter, 2021)

Sex for One: The Joy of Selfloving by Betty Dodson (Harmony, 2012)

Slow Pleasure: Explore Your Pleasure Spectrum by Euphemia Russell (Hardie Grant, 2022)

Want: Women's Fantasies in the Twenty-First Century edited by Gillian Anderson (Abrams, 2024)

"You Just Need to Lose Weight" and 19 Other Myths About Fat People by Aubrey Gordon (Beacon, 2023)

Relationships, Grief, and Healing

Books
All About Love: New Visions by bell hooks (William Morrow, 1999)

Decolonizing Nonviolent Communication, 2nd ed., by Meenadchi (Co—Conspirator Press, 2023)

Emotional Labor: The Invisible Work Shaping Our Lives and How to Claim Our Power by Rose Hackman (Flatiron Books, 2023)

It's OK That You're Not OK: Meeting Grief and Loss in a Culture That Doesn't Understand by Megan Devine (Sounds True, 2017)

Not That Bad: Dispatches from Rape Culture by Roxane Gay (Harper Perennial, 2018)

Sister Outsider: Essays and Speeches by Audre Lorde (Crossing Press, 2007)

Succulent Wild Woman: Dancing with Your Wonder-full Self! 25th Anniversary Edition by SARK (Atria Books, 2022)

With Pleasure: Managing Trauma Triggers for More Vibrant Sex and Relationships by August McLaughlin and Jamila Dawson, LMFT (Chicago Review Press, 2021)

The Wound Makes the Medicine: Elemental Remediations for Transforming Heartache by Pixie Lighthorse (Row House Publishing, 2023)

Domestic Violence Safety Planning

Domestic Violence Safety Plan
https://www.dvccct.org/wp-content/uploads/2020/03/Domestic-Violence-Safety-Plan-DVCC-.pdf

Checklist with hotlines to aid in escape, adapted from the Connecticut Coalition Against Domestic Violence's sample safety plan. Note that the National Domestic Violence Hotline is 800-799-7233; text 88788.

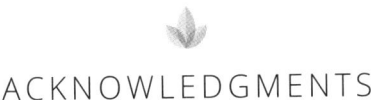

ACKNOWLEDGMENTS

Stephanie would like to thank:
Vanessa Carlisle, my co-author, is the one person who stands out when I think about this new edition. They are a jewel to work with and a kind, generous, thoughtful, intelligent, well-read, astute, and up-to-date colleague.

Penny Philpot. She has shared her wit, wisdom, patience, insight, and unconditional support for over thirty-two years. There are not enough words to express my appreciation and gratitude.

The many friends and colleagues who have encouraged and supported my work for decades.

Vanessa would like to thank:
First and foremost, Dr. Stephanie Covington has done more than she knows to uplift my work and, therefore, my self. Thank you for trusting me with this collaboration.

Max. For constant encouragement about writing, always being willing to hear difficult stories just before bed, and years of low-drama love after trauma.

J. The best hype-human in the world. Thank you for being my lifelong fambly, loving my work so deeply, and reminding me to take my own advice and be gentle with myself.

There is always a team.

We both would like to thank Roy Carlisle, who has influenced this book in several important ways. Stephanie is grateful to him as the developmental editor of the first version of *Awakening Your Sexuality* (1991) and also for introducing her to her co-author, Vanessa. Vanessa is grateful to Roy for being a parent who insisted that books were a necessity of daily life, and for introducing Vanessa to Stephanie.

We are both grateful to Andy Lien, our editor at Hazelden Publishing. She has supported this project from the beginning by advocating for its publication and providing thoughtful comments and ideas throughout the process.

We are both grateful to Elizabeth Gilbert, who offered so much insight, care, and time to this project.

We would also like to thank all of the authors, therapists, recovery group leaders, researchers, and activists who informed this book. Special gratitude to the women and nonbinary people in recovery who contributed their wisdom, words, and stories to this book.

ABOUT THE AUTHORS

Stephanie S. Covington, PhD, LCSW (she/her), is an internationally recognized clinician, organizational consultant, lecturer, and author in the fields of addiction and trauma. Dr. Covington serves as the co-director of the Institute for Relational Development and the Center for Gender and Justice. For nearly four decades, she has created gender-responsive and trauma-informed programs and services for use in public, private, and institutional settings. Author of the first manualized treatment program for substance use disorder treatment, Dr. Covington went on to create twelve trauma-informed, gender-responsive treatment curricula. Her most recent works include the 30th anniversary edition of the bestseller *A Woman's Way Through the Twelve Steps* and *Hidden Healers: The Unexpected Ways Women in Prison Help Each Other Survive*.

www.stephaniecovington.com
www.centerforgenderandjustice.org

Vanessa Carlisle, PhD, MFA (they/them), is an author, coach, and educator in the fields of gender, sexuality, and trauma. Dr. Carlisle's lived experience includes over twenty-five years in sex work and fifteen years of advocacy for the sex-working community. As a survivor of both intimate partner and institutional violence, Dr. Carlisle now crafts programs that combat stigma and improve conditions for their communities, including trauma-informed self-defense training, somatic coaching, and end-of-life care services. Along with many essays and articles, Dr. Carlisle authored the award-winning novel *Take Me with You* about a queer sex worker who must face her grief to be able to build the life she wants.

www.vanessacarlisle.com

ALSO BY THE AUTHORS

By Stephanie S. Covington, PhD, LCSW

Becoming Trauma Informed: A Training for Staff Development

Beyond Anger and Violence+: A Program for Women and Gender-Diverse People

Beyond Trauma: A Healing Journey for Women

Beyond Violence+: A Prevention Program for Criminal Justice–Involved Women

Exploring Trauma+: Brief Intervention for Men and Gender-Diverse People with Shane S. Pugh and Roberto A. Rodriguez

Healing Trauma+: A Brief Intervention for Women and Gender-Diverse People with Eileen M. Russo

Helping Men Recover: A Program for Treating Addiction with Dan Griffin and Rick Dauer

Helping Men Recover: A Program for Treating Addiction (criminal justice edition) with Dan Griffin and Rick Dauer

Helping Women Recover: A Program for Treating Addiction

Helping Women Recover: A Program for Treating Addiction (criminal justice edition)

Hidden Healers: The Unexpected Ways Women in Prison Help Each Other Survive

Leaving the Enchanted Forest: The Path from Relationship Addiction to Intimacy with Liana Beckett

Moving from Trauma-Informed to Trauma-Responsive: A Training Program for Organizational Change with Sandra L. Bloom

Voices: A Program of Self-Discovery and Empowerment for Girls with Kimberley Covington and Madeline Covington

A Woman's Way Through the Twelve Steps

A Woman's Way Through the Twelve Steps Facilitator Guide

A Woman's Way Through the Twelve Steps Workbook

Women and Addiction: A Gender-Responsive Approach

Women in Recovery: Understanding Addiction

A Young Man's Guide to Self-Mastery with Roberto A. Rodriguez

By Vanessa Carlisle, PhD

Take Me with You

A Crack in Everything

I Was My Mother's Bridesmaid: Young Adults Talk About Thriving in a Blended Family with Erica Carlisle

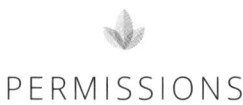

PERMISSIONS

The following publishers or authors have given permission to use quotations in this book from copyrighted works (in order of appearance):

Emily Nagoski, "My Lying Vagina, and the Lying Liars Who Lie About Her," February 20, 2016, https://enagoski.medium .com/everyone-is-lying-about-the-vaginas-77038767238d.

Adrienne Rich, *On Lies, Secrets, and Silence: Selected Prose 1966–1975* (W.W. Norton, 1995), p. 189.

Judith V. Jordan, "Clarity in Connection: Empathic Knowing, Desire, and Sexuality," Wellesley Centers for Women, Wellesley College, 1986, p. 6, https://www.wcwonline.org/pdf/previews /preview_29sc.pdf.

Meenadchi, *Decolonizing Nonviolent Communication*, 2nd ed., self-published by Co—Conspirator Press with the support of Women's Center for Creative Work, 2021, p. 41.

SARK, author of *Succulent Wild Woman: Dancing with Your Wonder-full Self!* 25th Anniversary Edition, personal interview.

adrienne maree brown, *Pleasure Activism: The Politics of Feeling Good*, AK Press, 2019, pp. 122–123.

ABOUT HAZELDEN PUBLISHING

As part of the Hazelden Betty Ford Foundation, Hazelden Publishing offers both cutting-edge educational resources and inspirational books. Our print and digital works help guide individuals in treatment and recovery, as well as their loved ones.

Professionals who work to prevent and treat addiction also turn to Hazelden Publishing for evidence-based curricula, digital content solutions, and videos for use in schools, treatment and correctional programs, and community settings. We also offer training for implementation of our curricula.

Through published and digital works, Hazelden Publishing extends the reach of healing and hope to individuals, families, and communities affected by addiction and related issues.

For information about Hazelden publications,
please call **800-328-9000**
or visit us online at **hazelden.org/bookstore.**